DRUGS AND NARCOTICS IN HISTORY

DRUGS AND
NARCOTICS
IN HISTORY

EDITED BY

ROY PORTER

Wellcome Institute for the History of Medicine,
London

AND

MIKULÁŠ TEICH

Robinson College, Cambridge

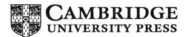

CAMBRIDGE
UNIVERSITY PRESS

Published by the Press Syndicate of the University of Cambridge
The Pitt Building, Trumpington Street, Cambridge CB2 1RP
40 West 20th Street, New York, NY 10011-4211, USA
10 Stamford Road, Oakleigh, Melbourne 3166, Australia

First published 1995
Reprinted 1996, 1998

Printed in the United Kingdom at the University Press, Cambridge

A catalogue record for this book is available from the British Library

Library of Congress cataloguing in publication data

Drugs and narcotics in history / edited by Roy Porter and Mikuláš Teich.
p.   cm.
Includes index.
ISBN 0 521 43163 8 (hardback)
1. Drugs – History.   2. Pharmacology – History.   I. Porter, Roy, 1946–
II. Teich, Mikuláš.
[DNLM: 1. Drugs – history.   2. Narcotics – history.
3. Drug and Narcotic Control – history.   4. Substance Abuse – history.
5. Drug Industry – history.   QV 11.1 D794 1994]
RM301.D789   1994
615'.1'09–dc20
DNLM/DLC for Library of Congress   94-20803 CIP

ISBN 0 521 43163 8   hardback

CONTENTS

vii

NOTES ON CONTRIBUTORS

CAROLINE JEAN ACKER is Assistant Professor of History at Carnegie Mellon University, Pittsburgh, Pennsylvania. She was formerly the first DeWitt Stetten, Jr, Memorial Fellow in the History of Twentieth-Century Biomedical Sciences and/or Technology at the National Institutes of Health, Bethesda, Maryland. She received her PhD from the University of California, San Francisco, in 1993 with a dissertation entitled 'Social Problems and Scientific Opportunities: The Case of Opiate Addiction in the United States, 1920–1940'.

VIRGINIA BERRIDGE is Senior Lecturer in History and Co-Director of the AIDS Social History Programme at the London School of Hygiene and Tropical Medicine. She has worked at the Addiction Research Unit, Institute of Psychiatry, the Institute of Historical Research, and the Economic and Social Research Council. She has undertaken consultancies for WHO-Euro and for the European Commission. Among her publications are *Opium and the People: Opiate Use in Nineteenth-Century England* (1981 and 1987) (main author); 'Health and Medicine 1750–1950', in *The Cambridge Social History of England* (1990); and *Drug Research and Policy in Britain: A Review of the 1980s* (1990) (as editor and author).

ANN DALLY is a psychiatrist. She read history at Somerville College, Oxford, then medicine at St Thomas's Hospital, London, qualifying in 1953. She became well known first for her work on mothers and children, then for opposing the 'official' treatment of drug addicts and the theories on which it is based. This got her into serious trouble with the General Medical Council (see her book *A Doctor's Story* (1990)). Her other recent books are *Inventing Motherhood* (1982) and *Women under the Knife* (1991). Since 1990 she has been working at the Wellcome Institute for the History of Medicine on fantasy surgery after Lister and, more recently, the history of some of the conflicts in psychiatry.

ERIKA HICKEL is Vice-President of the Technical University Braunschweig and Head of its Department for the History of Pharmacy and Science. Publications include *Arzneimittel-Standardisierung in den Pharmakopöen des 19. Jahrhunderts in Deutschland, Frankreich, Grossbritannien und den Vereinigten Staaten von Amerika* (1973); 'Emergence of Clinical Chemistry in the Nineteenth Century: Presuppositions and Consequences', in J. Büttner (ed.), *History of Clinical Chemistry* (1982); *Biochemische Forschung im 19. Jahrhundert* (1989) (as editor).

S. W. F. HOLLOWAY read medieval and modern history at University College London. He is interested in the history of the health care professions and has recently published a political and social history of the Royal Pharmaceutical Society of Great Britain. Most of his time is wasted trying to teach undergraduates at the University of Leicester.

STEPHEN J. KUNITZ is Professor in the Department of Community and Preventive Medicine at the University of Rochester, Rochester, New York. He received his MD from the University of Rochester in 1964 and his PhD in sociology from Yale University in 1970. He is the author of *Disease Change and the Role of Medicine: The Navajo Experience* (1983), *Disease and Social Diversity: The Impact of Europeans on the Health of Non-Europeans* (1994), and, with Jerrold E. Levy, *Drinking Careers: A Twenty-Five Year Follow-Up of Three Navajo Populations* (1994), as well as articles on the history of disease and on the sociology of medical knowledge.

JERROLD E. LEVY is Professor of Anthropology at the University of Arizona since 1972 and is co-author with Stephen J. Kunitz of *Indian Drinking: Navajo Practices and Anglo-American Theories* (1974) and *Navajo Aging: From Family to Institutional Support* (1991), and with Raymond Neutra and Dennis Parker, of *Hand Trembling, Frenzy Witchcraft, and Moth Madness: A Study of Navajo Seizure Disorders* (1987). He is also a former National Endowment for the Humanities resident scholar at the School of American Research. He lived for many years on the Navajo Reservation among the Navajo and Hopi Indians and has recently published *Oravvi Revisited: Social Stratification in 'Equalitarian' Society* (1992). He received his PhD in anthropology from the University of Chicago in 1959.

ANDREAS-HOLGER MAEHLE is a Wellcome Research Fellow in the History of Medicine at the University of Durham, England, and Privatdozent at the University of Göttingen, Germany. His publications include *Johann Jakob Wepfer (1620–1695) als Toxikologe* (1987) and *Kritik und Verteidigung des Tierversuchs: Die Anfänge der Diskussion im 17. und 18. Jahrhundert* (1992). He is currently working on a history of experimental pharmacology in eighteenth-century Britain.

RUDI MATTHEE holds a PhD in Islamic studies from the University of California, Los Angeles. He teaches Middle East History at the University of Denver. His area of expertise is early modern Iran, European expansion history, and modern Egypt.

JOHN PARASCANDOLA is Historian for the United States Public Health Service. He received his PhD in History of Science from the University of Wisconsin–Madison in 1968. After spending a postdoctoral year at Harvard University, he returned to Madison to join the Wisconsin faculty in history of science and history of pharmacy. In 1983 he became Chief of the History of Medicine Division of the National Library of Medicine, where he remained until moving to his current post in 1992. He is the author of *The Development of American Pharmacology: John J. Abel and the Shaping of a Discipline* (1992).

JOHN SCARBOROUGH is Professor of the History of Pharmacy and Medicine, and Professor of Classics, University of Wisconsin–Madison. He is the author of *Roman Medicine* (1969), *Facets of Hellenic Life* (1976), *Medical Terminologies: Classical Origins* (1992), and editor of the essay collections *Symposium on Byzantine Medicine* (1985) and *Folklore and Folk Medicine* (1987). He is also the author of several dozen essays in the professional journals on ancient Greek, Roman, Byzantine, and Arabic medicine, pharmacy, medical entomology, and related matters.

JUDY SLINN. Since reading PPE at St Anne's College, Oxford, Judy Slinn has researched into and written on business history and management. Her work on the pharmaceutical industry includes *A History of May & Baker 1834–1984* (1984) and, with Richard Davenport-Hines, *Glaxo: A History to 1962* (1992). Other publications include the histories of City law firms, Freshfields, Linklaters & Paines, and Clifford Chance. She teaches part time at Oxford Brookes University and is an Associate Editor on the new *DNB*.

ACKNOWLEDGEMENTS

AS EVER our special thanks are due to Frieda Houser from the Academic Unit of the Wellcome Institute for the History of Medicine and to William Davies of the Cambridge University Press for their help and support.

INTRODUCTION

ARE drugs a spectre that is haunting the world at the present time? This is a question which arises of necessity on reading headlines in newspapers such as these:

Drugs case shocks community. Sensational details of how a top scientist used his Cambridge laboratory to produce mind-bending illegal drugs instead of life-saving medicines have shocked the pharmaceutical industry.
Cambridge Evening News, 27 November 1993

It's the 'wonder drug' of the nineties, Prozac is an anti-depressant with a cultural identity of its own . . . Every successful drug generates controversy and none more than Prozac. Critics fear that it could herald a disturbing era of pharmacologically-induced social control of the kind visualized by Anthony Burgess in his novel Clockwork Orange. This may seem extreme, but Prozac is now being proclaimed not only as an anti-depressant but as a means of treating personality disorder of all kinds. At the same time it has inspired a spate of lawsuits from people alleged to have had bad experiences with it.
Guardian, 4 February 1994

We spend £1 billion on over-the-counter medicines for minor ailments each year. But are they actually doing us any good?   *Guardian*, 8 February 1994

Top-selling drug may have killed hundreds in Britain.
Sunday Times, 27 February 1994

Drugs belong both to nature and society and as such have diverse interactive dimensions, not least the historical one. There are assorted works treating sizeable aspects and phases of drug history but the subject, as this volume testifies, is one of growth. Here it is of value to observe that to take measure of drugs at present is of consequence for throwing light on their previous history. In the same way as to study the history of drugs is of import for comprehending their use and misuse in our times. To be sure the present-day situation cannot be compared with the one in the past either quantitatively or qualitatively:

I

There is a core of around 300 drugs that constantly appear in the medical documents, be they Greek, Latin, Chinese, or other ancient languages. Until the 19th century, there was a remarkable consistency about the drugs used and the resistance to changes in natural product drugs. A typical medicine chest of an 18th-century physician was not very different from a 13th-century physician's chest except the medieval physician would not have had the drugs from the New World, such as balsam of Peru, quaiacum, sasparilla and tobacco . . . The medicinal usage . . . of these substances, while known only as part of a plant, was discovered by folk medicine long before medicine and chemistry isolated the compounds.

In contrast many drugs are 'new' to modern times in another sense. By 1979, 80% of the twenty-five single ingredient drugs most frequently prescribed in the United States were introduced after 1950. One-half of them were introduced after 1960.[1]

Widely acknowledged, opium occupies in the history of drugs a distinctive position which is reflected variously in this collection. Thus Andreas-Holger Maehle shows that it was experimentation with opium, in the eighteenth century, that contributed vitally to the development of pharmacological and physiological thought. For one thing, it led to novel insights into the mode and site of drug action respectively: the idea of direct action through nerves gave way to the view of mediation – after absorption – through the blood circulatory system. For another thing, it was instrumental in distinguishing between conceptions of 'sensibility' and 'irritability', effectively laying the foundations for the development of modern neurophysiology and the study of muscle contraction.

To take another example from earlier times. In Classical antiquity, John Scarborough notes, familiarity with the danger of opium overdosage guided medical practitioners and patients to tread carefully. This leads him to conclude: 'Perhaps we should always put "addiction" in a context of interpretation, according to the social opinions which dominate a particular era.'

While the point is well made, it raises questions about the type of society which engenders specific ideas and policies about drug matters, how they come into being, are applied and change in time. The authors' concern with these issues, focusing upon a particular period and representative example, and teasing the debates and disputes around it, constitutes the unifying thread of the volume.

It is also demonstrated that the 'drugs' problem has a history – the standing of drugs (in all senses of the term) has often been highly contentious. Medical science has sought to unravel the properties (physiological, psychological, pathological) of potent substances. Users, the medical profession, public opinion, and the state have been involved in demarcating proper uses and approved users – processes that have often led to vehement conflicts. The boundary lines between use and abuse (by individuals, by medical professions, and by the pharmaceutical companies which, over the last century and a half, have increasingly been involved in developing, manufacturing, and marketing such substances, and so have a vast financial interest in them) have been powerfully contested. 'Alternative' medicine has sought to develop milder or more natural drugs. Clearly, these issues remain unresolved in the present day, when certain harmful and highly addictive substances remain freely available (alcohol, cigarettes). Some are available on doctors' prescriptions, and others are illegal, being the object of international contraband trades and the targets of 'drugs wars'.

What this historical collection underlines is that the scientific and technical developments in the drugs area, as elsewhere, are unstoppable. The question for human society is how to meet the challenge of a product such as Prozac. Awareness of the serious state of affairs is growing, as brought out by David Rothman (Professor of Social Medicine and History at Columbia University), that the resolution of the issue demands the wholesale transformation of society:

Today we stand and listen to Prozac; tomorrow we will listen to a new hormone, and the day after tomorrow, to a new genetic manipulation. I can conceive of strict rules and procedures, but I have great difficulty imagining them implemented and respected. We would need a very different breed of patient and doctor, and we would have to be a very different kind of society.[2]

NOTES

1 J. M. Riddle, 'The Methodology of Historical Drug Research', in his *Quid pro quo: Studies in the History of Drugs*, Variorum Collected Studies Series CS367 (Great Yarmouth, 1992), xv, pp. 1–19 (pp. 12–13).

2 D. Rothman, 'Shiny, Happy People', *Guardian*, 4 February 1994.

ONE

THE OPIUM POPPY IN HELLENISTIC AND ROMAN MEDICINE

JOHN SCARBOROUGH

WELL known from earliest Greek history,[1] the opium poppy (*Papaver somniferum* L.) occupied an important role in ancient pharmacy and medicine, and its use encompassed matters of dietetics as well as frequent employment as a soporific and general analgesic. Greco-Roman medicine and pharmacology incorporated a very succinct knowledge and command of the dangers and benefits in the use of the opium poppy, and actions of drugs were widely understood. Its harvesting, preparation, distribution, and application in general pharmacy and medical therapeutics all were sophisticated and as precise as was then possible. Our ancient sources attest repeatedly to this deep sophistication in the grasp and understanding of the opium poppy, and Hellenistic and Roman pharmacy had refined a lengthy and venerated tradition of multiple uses. Modern pharmacology and medicinal chemistry, of course, confirms much of this ancient expertise, even as we wrestle with the addictive effects of the major alkaloids commonly isolated and administered from the raw opium. One notes in the study of Hellenistic and Roman use of opium that the 'natural product' may have induced occasional addiction (and was certainly employed in suicides), but unlike the dangers explicit with the employment of morphine, codeine, thebaine, and other opium alkaloids in modern pharmacy and medicine, and ancients could presume their collected latex had benefits that far outweighed its dangers.

Homer's epics contain the first references in Greek literature to the opium poppy,[2] and one reads in the *Odyssey* that this drug is one which 'quiets all pains and quarrels'. One also hears that this beneficial substance is derived from a plant that grows in Egypt, a rather curious assertion since *Papaver somniferum* L. is native to Asia Minor, but a 'made in Egypt' label in Homer's day carried much medical weight. More curious is the lack of notice in our Greek sources of the opium poppy from Homer's time through the fifth century BC, and when Theophras-

4

tus considers *mēkōnes* in his masterful *Enquiry into Plants*,[3] there is but a brief notice of how one gathers the useful juice from the 'head' of the plant. In the Hippocratic corpus, there are thirteen references to the use of opium or the opium poppy,[4] and nine of these are nestled within the gynaecological tracts, suggesting employment among midwives but less frequent use by male physicians. In the Hellenistic Age, physicians were well acquainted with the dangers of opium poisoning, and added to the clipped references by Dioscorides[5] to the fears of the drug set down by Diagoras (*fl.* ?400 BC),[6] Andreas (d. 217 BC),[7] and Mnesidimus (*fl.* ?),[8] we have the rather accurate description of the results of fatal opium overdoses (and some antidotes) by Nicander of Colophon,[9] who lived in western Asia Minor about 130 BC. In the *De medicina* of Cornelius Celsus (*fl.* in the reign of Tiberius (AD 14–37)), one finds some possible references to the medical use of the latex of the opium poppy, but 'Celsus never alludes to the cultivated poppy from which opium is obtained', and since he '. . . does not include poppy juice in his list of poisons . . . he probably knew only a mild variety of the juice.'[10] Poppy tears (*lacrimae*) do figure in a number of Celsus' anodynes, but the source of these lozenges was probably the mildly narcotic *Papaver rhoeas*, not *P. somniferum*.

Dioscorides of Anazarbus (*fl. c.* AD 70) composed one of the most important works in all the history of medicine,[11] and his *Materia Medica*, IV, 64 (ed. Wellmann, II, pp. 218–21) contains the first and best summary of what the opium poppy 'did' in Hellenistic and Roman therapeutics. Dioscorides has used frequently various preparations of 'poppy-juice' in his own practice, extending over many years and several provinces in the eastern half of the Roman Empire. The traditions and practices recorded by Dioscorides throughout the *Materia Medica* often suggest clinical observations fused with folk medicine and a precise pharmacology, and it is what drugs 'do' when given to patients that occupies Dioscorides' major attention. Consequently, an organizing principle for the whole *Materia Medica* comes not through botanical morphology or an alphabetical listing of pharmaceuticals, but through what John Riddle has perceptively discerned as a 'drug affinity' system[12] – that is what happens when patients are given a particular drug or compound in the treatment of particular ailments. This is exactly the blueprint one meets in Dioscorides' account of the opium poppy: he begins with a general summary of where opium poppies grow (wild and cultivated), and proceeds with admirable clarity into general properties (in Greek *dynameis*) of the drug in its several forms, some special names applied to different kinds of poppies, preparation techniques, various applications in specific ailments, the detection of true opium from counterfeit lookalikes, and finally the most excellent description we have of the harvesting of the latex from the poppy capsules in Classical antiquity. In a departure, too, from his usual habits of not citing authorities from written works on pharmacology, Dioscorides suggests how earlier physicians had been quite in error in their fear of opium as an overly dangerous drug:[13] 'these very opinions are wrong, refuted through experience with the efficacy of the drug being observed in its results'. The names cited by Dioscorides – Erasistratus quoting Diagoras, Andreas, and Mnesidemus – indicate a debate and wide use of the opium poppy in medicinal pharmacy going back at least 400 years; it is little wonder that Theophrastus in his rightly renowned *Enquiry into Plants* does not emphasize the opium poppy among his limited listing of pharmaceuticals in Book IX,[14] since opinions among physicians and rootcutters varied so greatly. Comparison also with the accounts of opium in Pliny the Elder's *Natural History* to that in Dioscorides indicates some common sources of information (there is no evidence that Pliny knew the work of Dioscorides, or vice versa),[15] at least as such data were available on drugs from books; and to Dioscorides' list of written authorities on the opium poppy, Pliny adds Iollas, a name which appears in the *Preface* by Dioscorides to his *Materia Medica*.[16] Pliny designates 'the drug from the poppy capsule' in its Greek form, the *dia kōduōn*,[17] the term used continuously for this medicament from Pliny's day through the quotations in the works of Byzantine physicians.[18] In Galen's drug books, there is a list of embedded authorities on opium or the drug made from the opium poppy capsule,[19] and they range from Asclepiades and Themison,[20] to Damocrates' quoted poem *From the Poppy Capsule*,[21] a formula for the poppy capsule drug from the works of Soranus, mentions of similar formulas by Criton (physician to Trajan),[22] Heras,[23] and Galen's own version of the drug.[24] And with the exception of theriacs, as Galen relates the uses and properties of the opium capsule preparation, comparison with the text of Dioscorides reveals close parallels, showing that Dioscorides' explication incorporated the main lines of medical opinion on opium, accepted and followed by most learned physicians after *c.* AD 100. One can, therefore, take Dioscorides' *Materia Medica*, IV, 64, as representative of the best understanding in Hellenistic and Roman pharmacy of the properties, actions, and uses of the opium poppy. Dioscorides stands, moreover, in time on the bridge between Roman imperial medicine and the earlier heritages of Hellenistic practices, and his citations (for purposes of refutation) of Diagoras, Erasistratus, Andreas, and Mnesidemus give a glimpse of an earlier literature on pharmaceutical employment of the opium poppy and its latex.

Although Dioscorides was clearly a very skilled medical botanist, he spends few words on plant morphology, perhaps presuming that anyone interested in such matters would consult Theophrastus' very fine *Enquiry into Plants*. In beginning his section on the opium poppy, Dioscorides specifies that some varieties are 'cultivated and grown in gardens',[25] and that these garden poppies provide seeds made into a special bread recommended as particularly healthy by dieticians. The seeds of this garden variety poppy were also fit substitutes for sesame seeds, if the poppy seeds were mixed with honey, and this sesame seed replacement has the name 'common poppy' (Greek *thylaktis*),[26] with the plant bearing a white seed in a longish capsule. Dioscorides knew that poppy seeds had no narcotic properties, and his mention of white seeds from this cultivated type is strikingly verified by a modern description which notes that 'Seeds [are] used for preparation of emulsions (white-seeded varieties are preferred)',[27] even as poppy seeds 'contain no opium and are used extensively in baking and sprinkling on rolls and bread'.[28] Dioscorides' dietetic experts also knew how 'health-inducing' were these seeds, and modern food chemists have found goodly amounts of lecithin in poppy seed meal. It is significant that Dioscorides begins his section on the opium poppy with its dietetic uses, a signal not only of his organizational principles but also of the soon-accepted manner of compiling medical handbooks with initial chapters on healthy food-stuffs (usually plants) which also functioned as drugs.[29] And by commencing the account of the opium poppy with the garden variety, Dioscorides is suggesting two important aspects about Hellenistic and Roman understanding and use of the opium poppy: first, one can raise it in a garden for ordinary employment in the diet as bread and as a plant which yields a nourishing oil,[30] as well as some limited use as a narcotic; and, secondly, there is the assumption that uncultivated opium poppies provide the more potent latex, used almost exclusively as a drug. In speaking of the garden poppy, Dioscorides also includes two other kinds by way of introducing the more powerful varieties which will follow in the next section: there is a semi-wild poppy with a black seed called *pithitis* or *rhoias* – the corn poppy – so named 'from the latex (*opos*) flowing from it'; and a second kind is even less cultivated, which is smaller 'and more useful as a drug, having a longish capsule'.[31]

Turgidly Galen repeats[32] what Dioscorides had set down concisely 150 years previously regarding the properties of the opium poppy. In his usual terse and clipped manner, Dioscorides writes that 'a common property (*dynamis*) among [the kinds of poppies] is cooling',[33] and he proceeds immediately to say that the decocted leaves and capsules applied as fomentations bring on sleep. One may also drink this decoction for insomnia, but if the pharmacologist triturates finely the capsules and mixes this pounded poppy capsule in a poultice made from hulled barley and then formed into plasters, such a plaster could be used to treat inflamed boils (*phlegmonai*) and cases of St Anthony's fire (that is erysipelas). This is the weakest form of the drug, and its source is either a boiled down solution (here in water) or a combination of whole capsules and leaves with crushed barley, and Dioscorides' own experience with these preparations proved their usefulness in sometimes including slumber for insomniacs, and in successful treatment of skin problems, including reddened boils and the shiny and red lesions on the arms and legs or the face characterized by vesicles. Iranian folk medicine continues to employ for boils a paste made from compounded linseed (*Linum usitatissimum* L.), mallow (*Malva* spp.), and poppy,[34] and the modern pharmacopoeias record that the poppy capsule is mildly sedative.[35] And although opium does indeed have some bactericidal properties, one remains uncertain if Dioscorides' barley–poppy plaster would have been effective against the Group Λ beta-hemolytic streptococci causative of erysipelas, but it is probable that the mild analgesic itself alleviated the severe discomfort of patients afflicted by this superficial cellulitis.[36]

Immediately following his prescriptions for decocted poppy capsule and leaves, and the barley–poppy plaster, Dioscorides specifies another preparation technique for this mildly acting form of the drug: 'One ought to make it into lozenges – pounding them in a mortar while they are still green – and drying them to lay them up into storage, and thus employ it.'[37] Such lozenges, sometimes still called trochisks as borrowed directly from the Greek word, were easily stored and transported, and dried tablets retained their medicinal properties after they were remelted and used in plasters or in fomentations. It is in particulars like this that Dioscorides shows his practised experience with drugs, and parenthetically such specifics indicate that the best of the Greco-Roman physicians were also skilled pharmacists and compounders of drugs, as well as able medical botanists, quite capable of identifying plants in the field and gathering them for preparation as pharmaceuticals.

Next Dioscorides describes a slightly stronger form of the drug to be used as a 'pain-killing lozenge (*anōdynon ekleikton*) for coughs and tracheal discharges, as well as bowel conditions'.[38] The poppy capsules are to be boiled in water down to half the original volume, and then boiled again with honey until 'the moisture should condense out'. This process would give a syrup, which could be hardened into tablets, stored, and remelted for use as a Greco-Roman version of a cough medicine, or, sucked as would be modern cough drops, and gave the pain-killing remedy specified by Dioscorides. 'Poppy capsule . . . has been used as a liquid extract or syrup in cough mixtures',[39] showing that ancient applications of poppy for coughs have continued for two millennia. And as modern pharmacognosy texts repeatedly emphasize, 'Opium, while closely resembling morphine, exerts its action more slowly, and is therefore preferable in many cases, e.g. in the treatment of diarrhoea',[40] again a millennial-deep reflection of Dioscorides' recommendation that poppy capsules be used for 'conditions of the bowels'.

If one mixed *hyokistis* and *akakia* with the decocted honey–poppy capsule preparation, the compounded drug is 'more efficacious'[41] as a cough remedy and medicine for diarrhoea, and several other Roman writers agree with Dioscorides in recommending *hyokistis* and *akakia* for the control of both vomiting and diarrhoea.[42] The ever-cautious Soranus of Ephesus suggests the two in combination,[43] noting that these (among a number of substances) increase the effective properties of a 'styptic' or 'contracting action' (*stypsis*), that is what we would term adsorbent action in the digestive tract. The use of *akakia* in cough medicines is verified in modern practice: 'acacia is used as a demulcent in lozenges'.[44] *Akakia* is the famous 'gum arabic', the dried gum obtained from the stem and branches of *Acacia senegal* Willd., *A. arabica* Willd., and other species of *Acacia* in north and central Africa. Gum arabic's constituents explain – in modern terms – its well-known pharmaceutical properties, since it contains mostly arabin and the calcium salt of arabic acid along with traces of magnesium and potassium.[45] This natural combination makes gum arabic an excellent mucilage, tablet excipient, emulsifier, and thickener,[46] and adding *akakia* to the ancient version of the cough remedy made good sense in another way as well: Dioscorides has just mentioned putting the poppy capsule plus honey lozenges up for storage, and these trochisks would be employed later as needed; by adding and combining the opium poppy capsule and honey decoction with gum arabic, Greco-Roman pharmacologists were extending the effectiveness of the drug, or as the *Merck Index*, 11th edn, p. 11, notes, '[acacia is used] where flavor stability and long shelf life are important'.

Unlike the continued use of acacia in official medicine and pharmacy, the use of *hypokistis* had become 'obsolete' by 1830.[47] Well known to the Romans as an effective treatment for dysentery and milder forms of diarrhoea,[48] the juice of *Cytinus hypocistus* (L.) L., a member of the Rafflesiaceae (relatives of the mistletoe), has astringent properties and does retain a respected role in the folk medicine of southern Europe.[49] The modern pharmacopoeias do not include *Cytinus*, and there is little literature on its medicinal chemistry, but as a parasitic plant with bright yellow flowers growing from the roots of *Cistus* bushes (which produce balsams), it has been recorded clearly by Greco-Roman medical botanists in both its relation to the balsams and in its great usefulness in treatment of various diarrhoeas. As Dioscorides writes (perhaps quoting from Sextius Niger),[50] *hypokistis* has a property (*dynamis*) like that of *akakia*, but the *hypokistis* is 'more styptic and more drying'.[51] It appears that combining the *Cytinus* juice with gum arabic, and the decocted honey and poppy capsule preparation, would enhance the anti-diarrhoeal properties of this remedy, but as a therapy there might be some risk of constipation following milder cases of diarrhoea. Dysenteries are another matter altogether. Modern pharmacognosy does not detail why *Cytinus* has dropped out of use, even though folk medicine recognizes its value.

Perhaps the drying action of poppy seed oil engendered the belief that triturated poppy seeds quaffed in wine would alleviate diarrhoea and even hypermenorrhoea,[52] and the same assumptions appear to underlie the recommendation of applying a plaster of black poppy seeds with water to the forehead and temples to help insomniacs. Yet once Dioscorides has set down these ineffective suggestions, he tells us he is proceeding into data about the latex itself (*ho opos autos*), notably more cooling, thickening, and drying in its pharmaceutical properties than the poppy capsule preparations which have preceded: 'taken in as small a quantity as a bitter vetch seed, the latex is an anodyne and sleep-inducer, and it promotes digestion, being useful for coughs and intestinal conditions; but too much of the latex being drunk, it plunges one into lethargy in sleep, and it kills'.[53] Even as we read a reiteration of some uses of the opium poppy, met previously in the poppy capsule preparations, we also read that the latex by itself has fatal consequences if taken in too great a quantity. By citing the seed of the bitter vetch (*Vicia ervila* (L.) Willd. or *V. orobos* DC) as a 'unit of measure' or 'dosage', Dioscorides is making a very important point, well understood in Greco-Roman pharmacy: usually referred to in the plural in Greek, due to their small size, a seed of the bitter vetch by itself as a dosage unit would suggest the potency of such a measure of the opium poppy's latex, especially in an initial administration. Greco-Roman physicians were well aware that repeated use of raw opium (the latex) was – as we say – habit forming,[54] and that greater and greater dosages are required as time progresses to obtain the pleasurable effects, which include sleep accompanied by alluring dreams and visions.[55] Excessive and continued ingestion eventually leads to delirium and death, and as little as 300 mg of opium can be fatal to a human being[56] (it is on record, however, that some morphine addicts can tolerate 2,000 mg of morphine over a period of four hours). Approaching death is signalled by cold and clammy skin, a weak and rapid pulse, cyanosis, and (in modern diagnostics) pulmonary oedema, followed by a final pulmonary and circulatory failure.

Hellenistic and Roman medicine knew the dangers of the opium poppy's latex, and as early as the fifth century BC (if we have Diagoras' dates right) there was a firm opinion among physicians and pharmacologists that the opium poppy was in many instances too dangerous to employ as a drug. It is, however, in the hexameters of Nicander of Colophon (second century BC) that one initially gains a full view of Hellenistic recognition of opium poisoning, indicating lucidly enough how physicians and pharmacologists regarded the fatal potentials when someone quaffed too much of the 'tears of the poppy'.[57] Significantly, Nicander's verb is 'when they drink' (*pinōsin*),[58] showing that opium latex was well known as a drug in solution, and those who drink it 'fall completely asleep'. Also noteworthy is the similarity of Nicander's description of impending death to that given by modern physiological toxicologists:

their extremities are chilled; their eyes do not open but are bound quite motionless by their eyelids. With the exhaustion an odorous sweat bathes all the body, turns cheeks pale, and causes the lips to swell; the bonds of the jaw are relaxed, and through the throat the laboured breath passes faint and chill. And often either the livid nail or wrinkled nostril is a harbinger of death; sometimes too the sunken eyes.[59]

Nicander's suggested antidotes include hot wine, and the syrup made from grapes, as well as the oil of roses, olive oil, the oil of the iris, and slapping the hapless victim on the cheeks, shaking him too, hoping that vomiting will follow, 'ridding him of the fatal affliction'.[60]

A precious moment of Roman pharmacy is the *Compositiones* by Scribonius Largus, a tract that records what a well-versed physician–pharmacologist would recommend in the reign of Claudius (AD 41–54).[61] Opium latex (almost certainly *Papaver somniferum* L. in the recipes of Scribonius Largus) is a frequent ingredient in eye-salves (here *collyria*), ranging from gentle ones (*collyria lenia*),[62] to harsher ointments (*collyria acria*).[63] Scribonius' grouping of recipes for itch-salve (*collyrium psoricum*) includes two formulas containing opium latex,[64] and a Roman pound of opium is part of a six-ingredient drug applied in the treatment of nasal polyps.[65] Dehydrated opium figures in a compound drug for difficult breathing,[66] and many *catapotia* ('pills' here to function like cough drops) for coughs feature opium as a prominent constituent.[67] Scribonius prescribes opium much less for internal afflictions,[68] and there appears to be some caution perhaps inherited in part from his Hellenistic Greek medical texts, a caution in recommending opium for internal consumption. In the section titled *Ad opium*,[69] Scribonius follows the main lines already observed in Nicander's *Alexipharmaca* regarding the signs of opium poisoning (head becomes heavy, cold sweat, laboured breathing, deep sleep), and getting the person to vomit – using a feather or leather strap in the back of the throat – after forcing down some water mixed with oil is the first recommendation. Wine, vinegar, more oil, rose oil, more vinegar, and mustard follow in succession: one wonders, indeed, if the feet and legs plastered with a solution of mustard pounded in vinegar[70] would prevent the patient from falling back into sleep. Keeping the victim awake was essential.

By Pliny the Elder's day (the *Natural History* was dedicated to Titus in AD 77), an overdose was a common manner of committing suicide, as in the case of the father of Publius Licinius Caecina,[71] a senator during the short reign of Galba (AD 68–9). Pliny adds weightily to his tale of P. Licinius Caecina's father, *item plerosque alios* ('and thus also several others'), indicating that opium poppy latex was ordinarily available and occasionally used to end one's life *cum valetudo inpetilibus odium vitae fecessit* ('when an unbearable disease had rendered life hateful'). There is no mention of physicians or other medical specialists who might have been involved in procuring the opium, so one assumes the drug was sold openly and anyone could purchase it at one of the numerous druggists' stalls, where one could buy any medicament desired.[72]

Pliny and his sources, one of whom was Sextius Niger, also known and used by Dioscorides,[73] were observing the effects of the 'crude' opium latex, a complex mixture of 'at least 50 alkaloids, with the major constituent being morphine'[74] (morphine averages about 16%),[75] and the 'natural' combination provides a far different physiological and biochemical action in the body compared to one of the alkaloids acting alone. In fact, until Friedrich Wilhelm Sertürner isolated morphine from raw opium (his classic paper on the topic was published in 1817),[76] the observed physiological and pharmaceutical properties of opium resulted only from the combination of effects from the raw opium's multiple alkaloids. And in contrast to the lay person's assumption that opium latex (used in whatever form) is as potent as morphine or its laboratory-produced product heroin (made from morphine by replacing both hydroxyls with acetyl $-COCH_3$), a toxic dose of opium must be ten times larger than an equivalence of morphine for fatal effects.[77] Crude opium contains morphine (up to 20%), noscapine (up to 8%), codeine (up to 2.5%), papaverine (up to 2.5%), thebaine (up to 2%), and smaller amounts of narceine, protopine, hydrocotarnine, and the other alkaloids, as well as meconic acid (the fifty alkaloids are largely combined with this organic acid) and some lactic and sulfuric acid among other constituents including up to 25% water.[78] Raw opium's analgesic action results generally from its morphine, which acts directly as a depressant on the thalamus, the sensory cortex, and the respiratory and cough centres, but other alkaloids (especially codeine, papaverine, narceine, noscapine, and thebaine) have stimulant action on the medulla and the spinal cord; papaverine and noscapine, in particular, relax intestinal muscle, thereby providing a modern explanation of raw opium's use since antiquity in the treatment of diarrhoeas.

Hellenistic and Roman medicine had many salves and ointments enriched with ingredients presumed to have – in the modern terminology – transdermal action, and such remedies incorporating opium have continued to be used through the centuries, even though some modern authorities deny their effectiveness.[79] Cooling oil of roses mixed with opium poppy's latex was presumed to be a good headache remedy:[80] the latex and rose-oil were used as an embrocation, applied as would be the usual liquid medicament prepared for external use. The petals of *Rosa* spp., of course, are still utilized to produce the famous volatile oil (Attar of Rose, or Oleum rosae),[81] which remains important in the perfume industry. By the early twentieth century, however, rose-oil had assumed a minor role in pharmacy and medicine, becoming a 'grateful perfume' added to alcoholic preparations for internal use, as well as to wax-salves (cerates) and ointments. 'It is both too expensive and too powerful for most pharmaceutic purposes.'[82] Dioscorides also recommends opium poppy latex (again in liquid form),[83] in combination with almond-oil, saffron, and myrrh as a remedy for earaches: one pours or instils the mixture into the ear. As an eye-salve (or *collyrion*: a term not used here by Dioscorides), opium latex was combined with saffron and baked egg-yolk, and again one meets opium latex (this time in vinegar) as a treatment for erysipelas. For gout (the Greek literally says 'for pains in the feet'), opium latex joined with 'a woman's milk' and saffron was deemed effective as an external remedy. And as his last suggestion among the most useful applications of the opium poppy's latex, Dioscorides writes, 'And applied to a finger and used like a suppository, the latex induces sleep.'[84]

Almond-oil is derived from the seeds of *Amygdalus communis* L., and this fixed oil is an excellent vehicle for oily injections,[85] but almond-oil's major physiological action (as a mild laxative) is irrelevant here. Saffron is the dried stigmas of the styles of the saffron crocus (*Crocus*

sativus L.), and any drug – ancient or modern – which included this as
an ingredient would be costly: '100,000 flowers are needed to produce
1 kg of saffron.'[86] Saffron-oil (from the stigmas and petals) contains up
to thirty-four components, mainly terpenes, terpene alcohols, and
esters, and the effect of these constituents as part of an ear instillation
would combine with those of the opium latex. Opium tinctures with
saffron remain in the pharmacopoeias, and Sydenham's Laudanum (a
tincture made with opium, cinnamon, clove, and saffron) is listed in the
Martindale *Extra Pharmacopoeia*, 28th edn of 1982.[87] Modern pharmacology employs saffron in combination with opium (Sydenham's Laudanum is adjusted to contain 1% w/v of anhydrous morphine, with
recommended dosage of 0.25 to 2 ml), and it is probable that Greco-
Roman pharmacologists understood the benefits of combining saffron
with opium. It might be instructive to ascertain what pharmaceutical
properties are presumed in modern earache remedies, and one could
predict some parallels from ancient to modern.

The pharmaceutical properties of baked egg-yolk and human milk,
used as external applications, do not appear in the professional literature, although 'alum curds' (eggs beaten with alum) were commonly
employed as an astringent in the early twentieth century,[88] and a
milk-soaked piece of bread applied to a boil remains a favoured folk
remedy in many countries. Dioscorides' finger-coated opium suppository does, however, have its near-modern corollary: 'Suppositories of
opium with lead have been used to relieve rectal and pelvic pain, and
Gall and Opium Ointment is used for haemorrhoids.'[89] Modern literature and research on opium do not indicate any soporific effects, even
though Dioscorides and his sources are quite certain of this result.

Myrrh is, of course, the famous oleo-gum-resin collected as reddish-
brown lumps from natural cracks in the bark of *Balsamodendron myrrha*
(= *Commiphora myrrha* (Nees.) Engl.) and related species of what Majno
calls a 'scraggly, unfriendly tree of "crippled appearance"'[90] native to
north-eastern Africa and southern Arabia. Greco-Roman medicine
used myrrh in numerous manners,[91] but Dioscorides' ear-instillation of
myrrh as combined with opium, almond-oil, and saffron had observed
and reliable effects and benefits, especially if there chanced to be open
sores or wounds in the external auditory meatus. Myrrh in solution (the
lumps dissolve easily in water) is bacteriostatic against gram-positive
bacteria, including the most 'typical wound bacterium, *Staphylococcus
aureus*'.[92] If one considers the probable microbe-reducing properties in
saffron now fused with specificity against gram-positive bacteria, and
add the analgesic effects of opium, one ascertains what surely was a
useful drug for ear troubles. Again Dioscorides is prescribing opium in a

manner both cautious and helpful, and his combination of ingredients can elicit respect, even from modern pharmacologists. This short listing, moreover, of opium-remedies is all that Dioscorides recommends, indicating his care and painstaking observation throughout his career on what drugs 'do' and how they can be used safely.

Materia Medica, iv, 64. 5–7, takes up no further applications and uses of opium latex or any preparations of drugs from the opium poppy, but how to detect 'fake opium', followed by the short refutation of earlier Hellenistic authorities who had rejected opium in medical therapeutics; and finally (iv, 64. 7) is Dioscorides' description of how one harvests and prepares the opium poppy, both as a whole and as the latex alone; and if we recall that he has already specified an important 'when' for such harvesting – 'while [the poppy capsules] are still green' (*Materia Medica*, iv, 64. 2) – there is a hidden if very significant reason for this tradition of slitting or use of the whole capsule at this particular stage of its growth, a tradition 'explained' through modern chemistry. The centuries-old knowledge of the best time to harvest the latex, a knowledge gained by ancient farmers and botanists through a millennial trial-and-error, has received a remarkable confirmation from the study of biogenetics and phytochemistry.

The determination of the biogenesis of the opium alkaloids is, as one modern text puts it, 'a brilliant chapter in the history of phytochemical research'.[93] The first major alkaloid formed in the poppy capsule is thebaine, followed by an irreversible conversion to codeine, and then into morphine. The actual phytochemical process is, of course, far more complex than indicated by this simple summary, but one now perceives an answer to why ancient and modern harvesting of the opium latex occurs before the plant reaches full maturity. Ancient physicians and pharmacologists knew that the potency of opium latex had attained a certain level somewhat before the poppy capsule was fully ripened, and probably also understood that this particular level of potency suited medical employment within what we might call a margin of safety. One would welcome a future research project among phytochemists or pharmacologists which would demonstrate how much naturally occurring morphine is in the ripened poppy capsule: is the 20% morphine the greatest amount achieved (that is, the amount one finds when the capsules are slit while still green), or, is the more matured poppy capsule latex even more dangerous than the occasionally fatal substance widely utilized in Hellenistic and Roman medicine and pharmacy?

Comparison of harvesting techniques in a modern text,[94] with those given by Dioscorides in *c.* AD 70, shows little has changed over the centuries. Dioscorides' 'while still green' is a little more refined into when 'the colour is changing from green to yellow',[95] but even with more standard tools like scrapers, pan-receivers, and knives and multiple incision-makers,[96] there is little that marks a difference between modern Turkish or Indian latex gathering and the methods described by Dioscorides:

And it is not out of place to sketch out also the way in which they collect the juice [latex]; some, on the one hand, after beating the capsules with the leaves, squeeze it out through a press and pounding it in a mortar, they fashion lozenges: this as such is called *mēkōnion*, being less efficacious than the juice [latex]. But when extracting the latex, one ought to draw in the outline [*i.e.* cut] the 'little star' with a knife after the dew has evaporated, so that the incision does not perforate into the inside of the capsule, and to cut in from the top straight lines on the sides of the capsules, and to attach off the tear that comes out into a sea-mussel (*myax*) shell, and again to come back to this capsule after a short time; for there is to be found another congealed tear, and also another is to be found on the following day; one ought to pound it in a mortar and lay it up for storage when made into lozenges; and indeed in cutting the capsule for the latex one ought to stand back so that the latex is not attached to one's clothing.[97]

Drug fraud was common in Classical antiquity,[98] and detecting counterfeit opium was part of a physician's duty and skills. Dioscorides' methods are worthy of quotation in full, marked as they are by clarity and simplicity:

5. Best is the latex (*opos*) which is thick and heavy and soporific to the smell, bitter to the taste, easily diluted in water, smooth, white, neither rough nor full of lumps nor congealing as one passes it through [a sieve] as is [characteristic] of wax; set out in the sun and spreading, and being kindled by a lamp, it does not have a darkly coloured flame, retaining indeed its own particular odour. But they counterfeit it by mixing the juice of the horned poppy (*glaukion*) or acacia-gum (*kommi*) or the juice of the wild lettuce; that which is made from the juice of the horned poppy is like saffron in the solution, and that made from the lettuce loses its odour and is rougher, and that made from the acacia-gum is weak and translucent.
6. And some people are attended by so much madness so as to mix animal fat (*stear*) with it. And it is roasted in a new earthenware pot to make the eye-salves (*ta ophthalmika*) until it should appear soft and more tawny-orange.[99]

Modern opium remains an important item of illicit commerce, and it is not surprising that one finds the following in a contemporary reference on medicinal plants: 'The juice [of the horned poppy, *Glaucium flavum* Crantz] is used as a purgative, sedative and as an adulterant for opium',[100] and the gum from *Acacia* 'is light brown',[101] the latter showing why Dioscorides takes pains to write how the fake opium made from acacia is 'translucent' (*diaugēs*), and that the 'real stuff' is tawny-orange after roasting.

Finally, one can conclude with the role of opium in the famous theriacs of antiquity, especially the multi-ingredient drugs one reads in extensive quotation as given in the writings of Galen of Pergamon (AD 129–after 210). Much can be gleaned on the problems of theriacs and mithridatium in the book on the topic by Watson, but as a major ingredient of theriacs, opium is obscured in modern scholarship by assumptions that anyone who indulged regularly in opium-laced drugs would be as subject to addiction as twentieth-century dependants on heroin. In what may be a slip of the pen or perhaps rapid skimming of the texts of Galen – and finding what he expected to find – Watson writes 'Disconnected passages about Marcus [Aurelius] in [Galen's] writings, when pieced together, make a story of particular value, since it is the only case-record of a patron or addict of these fortifiers and remedies.'[102] That word 'addict' leaps out at any modern reader, and as such obliterates the context and sense of Galen's verbose account of exactly what the emperor Marcus Aurelius consumed and why he consumed it, presumably under Galen's direction.

Opium does figure as a major ingredient in the galene-poem by Andromachus the Elder,[103] and following the full quotation of this poem, Galen then lists the contents of a galene-formula by Andromachus the Younger which specifies 24 drachmas of opium.[104] A 'galene' to Galen is a broadly applied theriac: in addition to being a prophylactic against poisoning and the bites and stings of venomous animals, it was a kind of all-round, multi-ingredient preparation intended to promote a sense of well-being, comparable to modern anti-depressants (Andromachus the Younger's galene has just under sixty ingredients, with opium as number six, followed by oil of roses). Galen notes that he does, indeed, follow the formula of Andromachus (which of the two is not indicated) in his preparation of theriac (= ? galene) for the 'use of the royalty',[105] but Galen also writes that Marcus is taking as well a four-ingredient theriac (aristolochia, bitumen, rue, bitter vetch – to be taken in wine and oil (the drug first prepared as lozenges)) invented by Heras,[106] and there is no opium in the short formula.

Key passages on the question are in Galen's *Antidotes*, 1, 1,[107] and here one does read that Marcus Aurelius did consume daily the drug called Mithridatium in a dose measured to the size of an Egyptian bean.[108] And depending on whether Marcus wanted to sleep or to feel good about dealing with the day-to-day duties of being an emperor, the opium content was adjusted accordingly. Galen, moreover, points out that the emperor could distinguish high-quality theriac from that prepared from inferior ingredients,[109] suggesting not only that Marcus was well aware of particular effects from specific components but also that Galen shared with his royal patient exact and technical methodologies regarding the preparation of theriacs. Marcus Aurelius took his daily dose of Mithridatium with large quantities of honey,[110] and one can assume a 'sugar high' added to the elevated mood engendered by the opium in the theriac/galene.

One needs to recall that true addiction to opium requires greater and greater dosages to maintain the sensations of well-being,[111] and from the evidence teased from Galen's off-handed comments about how and when Marcus Aurelius used opium, the emperor was not addicted to opium. Marcus and his doctor knew exactly what they were doing and they used opium (among the many other ingredients in theriacs or galenes) carefully and with good control over physiological effects. One must infer from Galen's remarks that the emperor could 'cutback' on the opium as required in his function to perform his duties as ruler of the Roman Empire, and that on its own indicates Marcus Aurelius was not an opium addict. Perhaps we are afflicted with the negative nuances, currently in vogue regarding so-called 'addictive' substances, and one could easily make analogy to an 'addiction' (if so termed) to salicylates taken daily, even as physicians now recommend daily dosages of aspirin for the prevention of cardiac and vascular problems. Perhaps, too, as we peer and ponder the texts on opium and the anodynes commonly prepared from the latex of the opium poppy in Classical antiquity, we unwittingly reflect a common fear – exhibited by both lay persons and medical professionals – that opium's alkaloids are more dangerous than helpful. Physicians and their patients in Hellenistic and Roman times do not display this general unease, even as our shrewd ancestors were fully aware of the fatal consequences of opium overdoses. Perhaps we should always put 'addiction' in a context of interpretation, according to the social opinions which dominate a particular era.

NOTES

Unless otherwise specified, translations from the Greek or Latin are by the present author.

1 On this and related matters, see my 'The Pharmacology of Sacred Plants, Herbs, and Roots', in Christopher A. Faraone and Dirk Obbink, eds., *Magika Hiera: Ancient Greek Magic and Religion* (Oxford, 1991), pp. 138–74 (esp. pp. 139–42).
2 Homer, *Iliad*, VIII, 306–7; *Odyssey*, IV, 220–30.
3 Theophrastus, *Historia plantarum*, IX, 8. 2. See my 'Theophrastus on Herbals and Herbal Remedies', *Journal of the History of Biology*, 11 (1978), pp. 353–85.

4 E. Littré, ed., *Oeuvres complètes d'Hippocrate*, 10 vols. (Paris, 1839–61), x, p. 725 (index refs.: *pavot*).

5 Dioscorides, IV, 64. 6 = Max Wellmann, ed., *Pedanii Dioscuridis Anazarbei De materia medica*, 3 vols. (Berlin, 1906–14; repr. 1958), II, pp. 220–1.

6 In spite of Wellmann's confidence that Diagoras of Cyprus can be dated to the third century BC, there is great uncertainty regarding this physician, whose works are embedded in Pliny's *Natural History*, and against whom Dioscorides argues about opium. M. Wellmann, 'Diagoras (3)', in *Paulys Realencyclopädie der classischen Alterumswissenschaft* (= *RE*), v, pt 1 (Stuttgart, 1903), col. 311.

7 M. Wellmann, 'Andreas (11)', *RE*, I, pt 2 (Stuttgart, 1894), cols. 2136–7.

8 Dioscorides' citation of Mnesidimus is the single reference to this otherwise unknown Hellenistic physician, who appears to have been a noted authority on the opium poppy. K. Deichgräber, 'Mnesidemos (2)', *RE*, xv, pt 2 (Munich, 1901), col. 2275.

9 Nicander, *Alexipharmaca*, 433–64 = A. S. F. Gow and A. F. Scholfield, eds., *Nicander. The Poems and Poetical Fragments* (Cambridge, 1953), pp. 122–5.

10 W. G. Spencer, ed. and trans., *Celsus. De medicina*, 3 vols. (London, 1935–8), II, p. xlvi.

11 See John Scarborough and Vivian Nutton, 'The *Preface* of Dioscorides' *Materia Medica*: Introduction, Translation, Commentary', *Transaction and Studies of the College of Physicians of Philadelphia*, n.s., 4 (1982), pp. 187–227 (esp. 187–95).

12 John M. Riddle, *Dioscorides on Pharmacy and Medicine* (Austin, Tex., 1985), pp. 94–131.

13 Dioscorides, IV, 64. 6 (ed. Wellmann, II, p. 221).

14 Theophrastus, *Enquiry into Plants*, IX, 12. 4 = A. F. Hort, ed. and trans., *Theophrastus. Enquiry into Plants and Minor Works on Odours and Weather Signs*, 2 vols. (London, 1916), II, pp. 280–1.

15 See my 'Pharmacy in Pliny's *Natural History*: Some Observations on Substances and Sources', in Roger French and Frank Greenaway, eds., *Science in the Early Roman Empire: Pliny the Elder, his Sources and Influence* (London, 1986), pp. 59–85 (esp. 62 and 64).

16 Scarborough and Nutton, '*Preface* of Dioscorides' *Materia Medica*', p. 202.

17 Pliny, *Natural History*, xx, 200.

18 E.g. Oribasius, *Medical Collection*, v, 18–20 = J. Raeder, ed., *Oribasii Collectionum medicarum reliquiae*, 4 vols. (Leipzig, 1928–33), IV, pp. 132–6 (from the works of Galen and Philagrius).

19 Galen, *Compounding Drugs According to Place [on the Body]*, VII, 2 = C. G. Kühn, ed., *Claudii Galeni Opera omnia*, 20 vols. in 22 pts (Leipzig, 1821–33; repr. Hildesheim, 1964–5), XIII, pp. 38–47. In further citations, this edition of Galen's works will appear simply as 'K.,' with volume and page.

20 Asclepiades as cited may be Asclepiades of Bithynia (*fl.* in Rome *c.* 120 BC), but more likely Galen's source here is Asclepiades Pharmacion, a noted writer on drugs who lived in the reigns of Vespasian and Titus (AD 69–81). Cajus Fabricius, *Galens Exzerpte aus älteren Pharmakologen* (Berlin, 1972), p. 103. Galen, *Compounding Drugs According to Place*, x, 3 = K., XIII, p. 360, is a key passage for dating Asclepiades Pharmacion. Themison of Laodicea *fl.* in Rome under Augustus (31 BC–AD 14), and floats uncertainty as a 'pupil' of Asclepiades of Bithynia and one of the purported founders of the medical sect called

Methodists. For a cogent discussion of Themison's role in the development of Methodist theory, see now J. T. Vallance, *The Lost Theory of Asclepiades of Bithynia* (Oxford, 1990), pp. 141–2.

21 Galen, *Compounding Drugs According to Place*, VII, 2 = K., XIII, pp. 40–2. Servilius Damocrates *fl.* in the reigns of Nero and Vespasian (AD 54–79), and little of his writing is known except for quotations by Galen. M. Wellmann, 'Damokrates (8)', *RE*, IV, pt 2 (Stuttgart, 1901), cols. 2069–70. Fabricius, *Galens Exzerpte*, p. 189.

22 Soranus of Ephesus (*fl.* AD 98–117) wrote voluminously, but surviving in Greek are only his masterwork, *Gynecology*, and two shorter tracts *Signs of Fractures* and *On Bandages*, as well as a *Life of Hippocrates* = J. Ilberg, ed., *Sorani Gynaeciorum libri IV. De signis fracturarum. De fasciis. Vita Hippocratis secundum Soranum* (Leipzig, 1927). One knows of Soranus' writings on drugs solely through citations and quotations by Galen, E. Kind, 'Soranus aus Ephesos', *RE*, 2nd series, III, pt 1 (Stuttgart, 1927), cols. 1113–30 (esp. 1128–9). Criton (*fl.* AD 96–117) accompanied his royal patron on the Dacian campaigns, and became one of the ancient physicians who also wrote history. See my 'Criton, Physician to Trajan: Historian and Pharmacist', in John W. Eadie and Josiah Ober, eds., *The Craft of the Ancient Historian: Essays in Honor of Chester G. Starr* (Lanham, MD., 1985), pp. 387–405.

23 Heras of Cappadocia *fl.* in Rome *c.* 20 BC–AD 20, so Fabricius, 'Die Zeit des Heras' in his *Galens Exzerpte*, pp. 242–6. Quoted frequently by Galen, Heras investigated the properties of simples (Fabricius, *Galens Exzerpte*, pp. 209–12, lists the important ones), and became a widely used authority on drugs and compound medicines. Galen, *Compounding Drugs According to Place*, III, 1 = K., XII, p. 610, gives a formula for Heras' multiple-ingredient medicament 'For All Pains and Wounds in the Ear' quite similar to the recipe in Dioscorides, IV, 64. 4 (ed. Wellmann, II, 220). Heras includes the opium poppy, but adds frankincense to the portion of myrrh, and omits rose-oil, which Galen suggests one ought to reinclude (perhaps reflecting Dioscorides' formula).

24 Galen, *Compounding Drugs According to Place*, VII, 2 = K., XIII, pp. 43–5.

25 Dioscorides, IV, 64. 1 (ed. Wellmann, II, p. 218).

26 Cf. Galen, *Mixtures and Properties of Simples*, VII, 12. 13 = K., XII, pp. 72–4.

27 James A. Duke, *Handbook of Medicinal Herbs* (Boca Raton, Fla., 1985), p. 344. Paul G. Stecher *et al.*, eds., *The Merck Index*, 8th edn (Rahway, N.J., 1968), p. 850.

28 Duke, *Handbook*, p. 344.

29 E.g. Oribasius, *Medical Collection*, 1 = ed. Raeder, I, 4–27.

30 Cf. Duke, *Handbook*, p. 344.

31 Dioscorides, IV, 64. 1 (ed. Wellmann, II, pp. 218–19).

32 Galen, *Blendings*, III, 1 = G. Helmreich, ed., *Glaudius Galenus De temperamentis libri III* (Leipzig, 1894; repr. Stuttgart, 1969), p. 87. Galen, *Causes of Diseases*, III = K., VII, p. 14.

33 Dioscorides, IV, 64. 2 (ed. Wellmann, II, p. 219).

34 Duke, *Handbook*, p. 344.

35 R. G. Todd, ed., *Extra Pharmacopoeia Martindale*, 25th edn (London, 1967), p. 810.

36 *Ibid.*, p. 802, doubts the traditional use of opium liniments and lotions: 'There is no evidence of local analgesic action.'

37 Dioscorides, IV, 64. 2 (ed. Wellmann, II, p. 219).
38 *Ibid.*
39 James E. F. Reynolds and Anne B. Prasad, eds., *Martindale: The Extra Pharmacopoeia*, 28th edn (London, 1982), p. 1029 (No. 6260-y).
40 E.g. George Edward Trease and William Charles Evans, *Pharmacognosy*, 11th edn (London, 1978), p. 576.
41 Dioscorides, IV, 64. 2 (ed. Wellmann, II, p. 219).
42 E.g. Pliny, *Natural History*, XXVI, 49; Galen, *Affected Parts*, II, 9 = K., VIII, p. 114). Cf. Dioscorides, I, 97 (ed. Wellmann, I, pp. 87–9).
43 Soranus, *Gynecology*, I, 50. 3 (ed. Ilberg, p. 36).
44 Reynolds and Prasad, eds., *Martindale*, p. 949 (No. 5402-m).
45 William Charles Evans, *Trease and Evans' Pharmacognosy*, 13th edn (London, 1989), p. 373.
46 Susan Budavari *et al.*, eds., *The Merck Index*, 11th edn (Rahway, N.J., 1989), p. 11 (No. 10).
47 Wolfgang Schneider, *Lexikon zur Arzneimittelgeschichte*, 7 vols. in 9 parts (Frankfurt, 1968–75), V, pt 1, p. 419.
48 Dioscorides, I, 97. 2 (ed. Wellmann, I, pp. 87–8). Galen, *Mixtures and Properties of Simples*, VII, 10. 27 = K., XII, 27–8.
49 Oleg Polunin, *Flowers of Europe* (London, 1969), p. 61.
50 So Wellmann in apparatus criticus to line 10, Dioscorides, I, 87.
51 Dioscorides, I, 97. 2 (ed. Wellmann, I, p. 88).
52 Dioscorides, IV, 64. 3 (ed. Wellmann, II, p. 220).
53 Dioscorides, IV, 64. 3 (ed. Wellmann, II, p. 219).
54 Pliny, *Natural History*, XX, 199.
55 Albert F. Hill, *Economic Botany*, 2nd edn (New York, 1952), p. 279.
56 Duke, *Handbook*, p. 345.
57 Nicander, *Alexipharmaca*, 433.
58 *Ibid.*, 434.
59 *Ibid.*, 434–42. The translation is by Gow and Scholfield, *Nicander*, p. 123.
60 Nicander, *Alexipharmaca*, 460.
61 Sergio Sconocchia, ed., *Scribonii Largi Compositiones* (Leipzig, 1983), pp. vi–vii. Scribonius Largus accompanied Claudius in the Roman invasion of England in AD 43.
62 *Ibid.*, pp. 19–27.
63 *Ibid.*, pp. 28–31.
64 *Ibid.*, pp. 32 and 33.
65 *Ibid.*, p. 52.
66 *Ibid.*, p. 77.
67 *Ibid.*, pp. 85–93.
68 E.g. *ibid.*, pp. 112, 115, and 120.
69 *Ibid.*, p. 180.
70 'sinapi ex aceto tritum circumdatum pedibus cruribusque et a somni tempore prohibere'.
71 Pliny, *Natural History*, XX, 199–200. Tacitus, *Histories*, II, 53.
72 Pliny, *Natural History*, XXIV, 108.
73 Scarborough, 'Pharmacy in Pliny's *Natural History*', p. 67.
74 George Lenz *et al.*, *Opiates* (Orlando, Fla., 1986), p. 2.

75 Budavari *et al.*, eds., *Merck Index*, p. 6810 (No. 6809).

76 Ronald D. Mann, *Modern Drug Use. An Inquiry on Historical Principles* (Boston, Mass., 1984), p. 471.

77 Todd, ed., *Martindale*, p. 801.

78 Budavari *et al.*, eds., *Merck Index*, p. 6810 (No. 6809) with refs.

79 E.g. Todd, ed., *Martindale*, p. 802 (opium).

80 Dioscorides, IV, 64. 4 (ed. Wellmann, II, p. 220).

81 Trease and Evans, *Pharmacognosy*, p. 411.

82 Horatio C. Wood, Charles H. LaWall *et al.*, *The Dispensatory of the United States of America*, 22nd edn (Philadelphia, 1937), p. 773.

83 Dioscorides, IV, 64. 4 (ed. Wellmann, II, p. 220).

84 *Ibid.*

85 Trease and Evans, *Pharmacognosy*, p. 313.

86 George Usher, *A Dictionary of Plants Used by Man* (London, 1974), p. 183.

87 Reynolds and Prasad, eds., *Martindale*, p. 1022.

88 Wood and LaWall *et al.*, eds., *Dispensatory*, p. 805.

89 Todd, ed., *Martindale*, p. 802; dropped from *Martindale*, 28th ed.

90 Guido Majno, *The Healing Hand, Man and Wound in the Ancient World* (Cambridge, Mass., 1975), p. 212.

91 *Ibid.*, pp. 215–17, with refs.

92 *Ibid.*, p. 217.

93 Trease and Evans, *Pharmacognosy*, p. 561.

94 Evans, *Trease and Evans' Pharmacognosy*, p. 583.

95 Trease and Evans, *Pharmacognosy*, p. 570.

96 *Ibid.*, p. 571, with Fig. 170.

97 Dioscorides, IV, 64. 7 (ed. Wellmann, II, pp. 221).

98 See esp. Vivian Nutton, 'The Drug Trade in Antiquity', *Journal of the Royal Society of Medicine*, 78 (1985), pp. 138–45.

99 Dioscorides, IV, 64. 5–6 (ed. Wellmann, II, p. 220).

100 Usher, *Dictionary*, p. 275.

101 *Ibid.*, p. 12.

102 Gilbert Watson, *Theriac and Mithridatium* (London, 1966), p. 87.

103 Galen, *Antidotes*, I, 6 = K., XIV, pp. 32–42, esp. line 121 of the poem. Andromachus the Elder was physician to Nero (AD 54–68), and his son, Andromachus the Younger, also functioned as a court doctor in the reign of Nero. Fabricius, *Galens Exzerpte*, pp. 185–6.

104 Galen, *Antidotes*, I, 7 = K., XIV, pp. 42–4, esp. 42.

105 Galen, *Theriac to Piso*, 12 = K., XIV, p.262.

106 Galen, *Antidotes*, II, 17 = K., XIV, p. 201.

107 K., XIV, pp. 3 and 5.

108 Galen, *Antidotes*, I, 1 = K., XIV, p. 4.

109 Galen, *Antidotes*, I, 1 = K., XIV, p. 5.

110 Roman medicine included honey as a potent drug, employed in numerous manners, as one reads in many passages and sections of Galen's writings, e.g. *Mixtures and Properties of Simples*, VII, 12. 9 = K., XII, pp. 70–1. Dioscorides, II, 82 (ed. Wellmann, I, pp. 165–7) is probably the most concise summary of pharmaceutical properties, as understood in Hellenistic and Roman pharmacy. What

Dioscorides terms *sakcharon* in II, 82. 4 (Wellmann, I, p. 167) is, incidentally, one of our first references to sugar cane from India.

111 A classic description remains that in Solomon Solis-Cohen and Thomas Stotesbury Githens, *Pharmacotherapeutics* (New York, 1928), p. 263.

TWO

EXOTIC SUBSTANCES: THE INTRODUCTION AND GLOBAL SPREAD OF TOBACCO, COFFEE, COCOA, TEA, AND DISTILLED LIQUOR, SIXTEENTH TO EIGHTEENTH CENTURIES

RUDI MATTHEE

INTRODUCTION

FROM the late sixteenth to the early eighteenth century substances with addictive qualities such as tobacco, coffee, cacao, tea, and distilled liquor were introduced, found acceptance, and spread with remarkable speed around the globe.[1] The near-simultaneity of the introduction and the similarity in the reception and dissemination of these psychotropic substances among the population of Europe and parts of America, Asia, and Africa is striking enough to invite comparisons. To draw such comparisons is the aim of the following discussion, which will consider the transformation of these five stimulants from curiosity and rarity to commonplace commodity in the context of a number of converging and intersecting economic, social, and political processes.

The first of these is the expansion of European horizons in the wake of the great maritime discoveries at the turn of the sixteenth century. Europe's exploration of the globe not just ushered in a commercial revolution, but simultaneously helped ignite a revolution in scientific and religious thought and practice that was to have a lasting impact on the world. While the Renaissance overturned the existing canons of science and philosophy and inspired a new focus on the physical and the material, the Reformation forced a new consciousness upon man, urging him to contemplate God individually and to conduct his life according to a new personal ethic. In the practical morality of subsequent movements such as Puritanism and Pietism the new stimulants became indices of individual responsibility, and were alternately denounced as emblems of moral rot and social degeneracy, or celebrated as the embodiment of sobriety and vigilance.

The individualization of society adumbrated by Renaissance and Reformation occurred in the context of the second process, the rise of the early modern state. Built around new bureaucratic structures, legitimized through institutionalized religion, and relying on standing armies, sixteenth- and seventeenth-century states everywhere formulated centralist commercial policies and advanced claims to regularized taxation. While at first the relevance of the exotic wares was limited to mercantilist preoccupations with the balance of trade, this changed as soon as governments began to recognize their value as taxable commodities.

Great new urban centres in western Europe formed the loci of this new political configuration. Their expansion spawned new commercial and administrative elites as well as a rudimentary urban proletariat, and redefined the boundaries between private and public spheres. The growing social stratification and the segregation of class and gender inherent in this development marks the third and final process to be examined for its particular effect on the status of the new substances and the ambience in which they were consumed.

The following discussion will consider four aspects of the stimulants as they pertain to the processes just outlined. First a brief survey will be given of their expansion beyond Asia and South America. This will be followed by an examination of the similarities in early perception. Next the controversy surrounding the new stimulants in many parts of the world will be discussed. Lastly, the question of their wider dissemination and popularization will be considered. In all cases the written sources happen to be most abundant for Europe; much of the discussion will therefore inevitably centre on that continent. Throughout, however, the widest possible geographical scope will be considered and, wherever possible, parallels will be drawn with other parts of the world.

ORIGINS AND INTRODUCTION

The age of discovery and the subsequent trade expansion provides the backdrop to the introduction of all but one of the stimulants under discussion. Good examples are tobacco and cacao, both of which were introduced in the wake of the early European colonization of the Americas. Tobacco is generally held to have been introduced from the Caribbean and Brazil by the early European discoverers. Whether or not the tobacco plant and its use were unknown to any civilizations outside the western hemisphere prior to 1492, the fact is that the first Europeans to witness tobacco smoking were members of Christopher Columbus' crew.[2]

The knowledge and sporadic use of tobacco remained confined to the Mediterranean world for the next half century, but spread quickly after that. Theoretical knowledge advanced through works such as the popular *Agriculture et maison rustique*, a book on horticulture by Jean Liebault, and the *Cruydeboeck*, written by the Flemish Rembertus Dodonaeus in 1554 and held to be the oldest reference to the cultivation of tobacco in Europe.[3] Jean Nicot, whose name is immortalized in the addictive substance in tobacco, contributed to the early knowledge by describing tobacco while he served as the French ambassador to the Portuguese crown in 1560.

The first group to use tobacco in Europe were the soldiers and sailors who set out on military expeditions and commercial ventures from the ports of Lisbon, Genova, and Naples. Trade took tobacco further north. In the late sixteenth century those who would later become the chief distributors around the world, the English, took up smoking. The first clay pipes, modelled after Indian examples, began to be manufactured in London in about 1580. Sailors and travellers brought the tobacco habit from Portugal and England to Holland, and further on to Norway, where tobacco appeared in the import duty tariffs in 1589.[4]

War and commerce similarly furthered the spread beyond Europe's coastal regions. The Thirty Years War disseminated tobacco into central Europe, where English troops put at the disposal of Frederick of Bohemia in 1620 were seen smoking as they marched through Saxony. Before long, Germany was cultivating its own tobacco and served as a springboard for the spread to Austria and Hungary.[5]

Further afield tobacco was introduced through commercial channels. English merchants introduced tobacco to Russia in the 1560s. In Africa and Asia tobacco penetrated by way of Portuguese and Dutch sailors and merchants. Smoking was reported in Sierra Leone as early as 1607, while southern Africa was exposed to tobacco with the Dutch founding of the Cape colony in 1652.[6] In most of Asia tobacco penetrated in two ways. Central Asia acquired the tobacco habit via Iran, which, in turn, had come into contact with it through Portuguese commerce and Ottoman military campaigns. Japan, on the other hand, learned of smoking directly from the Portuguese. Tobacco probably spread to Korea and Manchuria with the Japanese occupation of the Korean peninsula at the same time that it was introduced in southern China by the Portuguese from Macao.[7]

A second substance whose introduction in the Old World resulted from the discovery of the New World is cacao. Cocoa, the drink prepared from cacao beans, originally was consumed as a spicy beverage, *xocoatl*, by the Indians of the Amazon basin, Venezuela, and Mexico. The beans were among the specimens Columbus brought back from his exploratory voyage. The first assortment shipped to Spain was seen as useless, however, and discarded.[8] Hernan Cortés, the conqueror of Mexico, was the next European to learn of cacao; he reintroduced the bean as well as the knowledge of its application to the Iberian peninsula, where it was kept a secret during the entire sixteenth century. Aside from occasional shipments to Spain, most of its trade until the early 1700s remained confined to traffic between Venezuela and Mexico.[9]

While tobacco and cacao travelled from west to east, coffee went in the opposite direction and was introduced in Europe from the Ottoman Empire via trade and travel. Coffee, which is now acknowledged to have originated in Ethiopia, from where it spread to Yemen, became known and found its way to other parts of the Middle East, particularly Egypt, via the Red Sea trade beginning in the fifteenth century, 200 years prior to its introduction in Europe. Coffee was known in Cairo by 1510, and the first coffeehouse in Damascus opened in 1530. The Turkish conquest of Mesopotamia facilitated the further spread from the Fertile Crescent across the Ottoman Empire: in 1554 the inhabitants of the capital Istanbul were able to savour the new drink.[10] Other parts of West Asia soon followed. Neighbouring Safavid Iran, for instance, must have been introduced to coffee within decades after its spread in Turkey, for by the early seventeenth century a number of bustling coffeehouses lined the main square of its capital Isfahan.[11]

Europe was soon to learn of coffee as well. The first European to taste coffee may have been the German physician Leonhard Rauwolf, who learned of it in Aleppo in 1573.[12] It was not much later, in 1592, that coffee was included as an entry in the herbal treatises of the Italian physician Prosper Alpinus.[13] Almost half a century later the drink itself made its appearance in Europe, where it was introduced to Italy and France by Venetian and Armenian merchants. Coffee was sold in Venice in 1640. In France, Marseille had its first acquaintance with coffee in 1644 and Paris soon followed suit. The first European coffeehouse opened in Venice in 1645.

Simultaneously, coffee began to be imported via the maritime trade. The Dutch, whose trade records from Mokha mention coffee beans in 1616, were the first Europeans to include coffee in their commercial activity.[14] The Dutch East India Company (VOC, for Verenigde Oostindische Compagnie) for decades confined coffee to its intra-Asian network.[15] It was only in 1661, more than twenty years after the Amsterdam Chamber of the VOC had ordered a first sample, that the home country received its first substantial supply.[16]

The earliest western mention of tea, which originated in China and had long been known in East Asia, is found in a work from 1559 by the Venetian author and administrator Giambatista Ramusio. Slightly later references occur in the correspondence of the Portuguese missionaries da Cruz and Almeida.[17] Despite these early accounts, however, a wider knowledge of tea in Europe had to wait for the establishment of the maritime companies. In 1607 the VOC shipped its first tea from Macao to Bantam; three years later Holland received its first shipment.[18] The earliest written reference to tea in the English East India Company (EIC) records dates from 1615.[19] But it was, after a ceremonial order in 1664, only in 1668 that the company placed its first public tea order directly from the east.[20] As well as via transshipment from China, the leaves also reached Europe via the land route between the Far East and Moscow, which became operative at approximately the same time that the west received its first maritime supplies.

Alcohol had of course been known in Europe from antiquity. From the barley drink of Sumeria to the wine in Greece and Rome and the beer of the medieval monasteries, alcohol had long been associated with religious ritual, economic enterprise, and social gathering. Tenth-century Muslim alchemists experimented with the distillation of alcohol, but only in early twelfth-century Europe does the perfect chemical separation of alcohol seem to have been performed. The large-scale introduction and consumption of distilled liquor had to wait yet longer: it did not occur in most of Europe until the late sixteenth and early seventeenth centuries. In Ireland, whiskey was a popular drink as early as 1550, but in wine-drinking France and ale-drinking England the spread of spirit drinking was much slower. France began to manufacture cognac in the 1630s, when distillers and sellers were also organized in a guild. In England spirit consumption took off in the mid-seventeenth century, mainly as a result of the ever-rising duty on beer. In Holland, where the first distillery was established in 1575, a surge in trade and prosperity as well as technological change soon spawned a phenomenal growth of the industry.[21]

Spirits caught on early in Russia as well. While it is unclear exactly when vodka made its entry into Russian social life, it is likely that spirits were first introduced by foreign mercenaries in the first half of the sixteenth century. This would seem to be confirmed by the institution of the state-controlled drink-shop (*kabak*) by Tsar Ivan in the middle of the same century.[22] In these saloons distilled spirits – mostly vodka – gradually displaced other beverages such as mead, kvass, and beer.[23]

EARLY PERCEPTIONS

Remarkable similarities are found in the way early modern society perceived and debated the new substances upon their introduction.

Without exception, initial classification and description occurred not under the heading of food, beverages, or entertainment, but that of medicinal agents. The context was the rapid transformation of the foundation of scientific enquiry in post-medieval Europe, where the canon of antiquity and the reasoning intellect began to guide the pursuit of science, and experimentation gradually replaced deference to transmitted knowledge. Botany, alchemy, and medicine were among the sciences thus affected. Modern botany emerged from a commingling of the medieval herbal tradition, a new interest in the classics, and the influx of living samples of new plants and exotic crops, all of which gave rise to the systematic analysis and classification of plants.

An incipient medicalization of society was another outcome of the same process. As experimental research into bodily properties and functions slowly began to undermine the Galenic humoral pathology that had long dominated medical thinking, new theories were developed about the working of the human body, the cause of ailments, and their remedies. In the resulting quest for experimental material and curative agents the new stimulants played a prominent role.

Tobacco was one of the substances that aroused lively botanical interest. Commissioned to study the indigenous flora and record new species of plants, botanists early on joined the Spanish adventurers to the New World. Thus, the private physician of Philip II, Hernandez de Toledo, who was sent to Mexico in 1559 to study the local flora, brought tobacco plants back to Spain, where they were subsequently cultivated in the royal gardens.[24] The title of Dodonaeus' work – *Cruydeboeck*, Book of Herbs – clearly indicates the category into which tobacco fell for the seventeenth-century European scholar. The chapter devoted to tobacco lists a long series of ailments against which it was held to be effective. Tobacco seeds and leaves are credited with healing powers for afflictions as varied as running wounds, whitlow, rashes of the face, scrophulus, and rabies. The author further pays a great deal of attention to the medical applications of nicotine, prescribing it as a remedy for injuries of head, arms, and legs, which must be washed with wine or urine prior to treatment with the leaves or the juice of the tobacco plant.[25]

Tobacco quickly became known as a panacea. Its exotic aura explains its early seventeenth-century renown as an aphrodisiac and may have contributed to its vaguely sacral and magical connotations in the early stages of introduction. More practically, tobacco was considered to be a disinfectant in a time in which frequent outbreaks of the plague left people desperate for preventive medicine. Praised as such during the 1635–6 epidemic in Holland, tobacco maintained that reputation during the 1665 plague of London and the epidemic that afflicted Vienna in 1679.[26] Those who brought tobacco back from the New World also claimed that it was capable of curing a disease they had carried with them from the Americas as well – syphilis. Others held that the substance was effective against thirst, hunger, and insomnia.[27] In India tobacco appears to have been used against tooth-ache and scorpion bites.[28] European popular imagery, finally, depicts Jean Nicot presenting tobacco to Catherine de Medici as a remedy against her migraine. Not surprisingly, the first to make commercial use of tobacco were apothecaries.

A candidate only slightly less likely than tobacco nowadays to be seen as a healing agent is cacao. Yet the beans of the cacao plant, too, were credited with medicinal qualities in the early phase of their introduction in the west. Europeans claimed that the Indians considered the spicy chocolate drink made from cacao to be good for the stomach and a cure for catarrh. The Aztecs did indeed use cocoa as a medicine against diarrhoea and dysentery and also considered it an aphrodisiac. This latter attribute, which was common to many newly introduced exotic products, crossed over to Europe, where in elite circles cocoa acquired an aura of erotic refinement.[29]

Europeans were slow in getting used to the bitter taste of the new drink, which was taken cold and blended with chillies and other spices. The English physician Henry Stubbe, who wrote a treatise on chocolate for a curious doctor friend in Oxford, noted that its taste was considered 'bitterish and adstringent' and 'none of the most pleasant to those that are not used to it'.[30] He nevertheless sang chocolate's praises as a wholesome beverage, noting its nourishing quality, its capacity to 'allay splenetique fumes and drowsiness', to 'generate good blood', and to promote 'natural expurgation'.

Coffee and tea were two more exotic substances which Europeans initially valued as medicinal agents rather than as ingredients of tasty beverages. Coffee beans were long sold by grocers and spice dealers as a drug. Thomas Herbert called coffee 'more wholesome than toothsome', and cited its reputation as a substance that 'confronts raw stomachs, helps digestion, expels wind, and dispels drowsiness'.[31] A generation later, Philippe Dufour, drawing attention to its capacity to render blood 'less acrid and more fluid', noted that doctors prescribed coffee for women during menstruation and after childbirth.[32] Not surprisingly, VOC records refer to coffee as 'that medicine'.[33]

In England, where it was perceived similarly in the seventeenth century, coffee won the sympathy of the famous physician William Harvey, who praised its medicinal qualities. Coffee indeed became widely prescribed by doctors, many of whom saw it as a welcome antidote to alcoholism.[34] This latter property, as well as its reputed anti-aphrodisiacal effect, accounts for the grudging approval coffee was given by the Puritans. For their part, the owners of the newly opened coffeehouses were naturally quick to advertise the outlandish concoction as a cure for a wide array of diseases.

As Galenic notions dominated Islamic as much as Christian medicine, it is not surprising to find that the authors of sixteenth- and seventeenth-century Arab and Persian medical and botanical manuals perceived coffee in much the same way as their European counterparts. Discussing the properties of coffee, they stressed its coldness and dryness; in their enumeration of remedial qualities they listed gastric and respiratory ailments; while among the negative humoral effects of overindulgence they mentioned haemorrhoids, headaches, and a reduced libido.[35]

Tea quickly acquired the therapeutic image it has retained until today. In England, early coffeehouse proprietors advertised the new drink to unfamiliar customers as a novelty 'approved by all physicians'.[36] The French Cardinal Mazarin drank tea against his gout.[37] In late seventeenth-century Russia, too, tea was consumed mainly for medicinal purposes: many drank it before or after indulging in liquor.[38]

No one, however, did more to make tea respectable than the physicians of the empirical medical school that emerged in the enlightened Dutch Golden Age. Substituting a contrast between salutary and unhealthy for the traditional good versus evil dichotomy, its representatives, prominent doctors like Nicolaas Tulp and Stephan Blankaart, adumbrated the secularization of medicine. Tea was one of the substances they studied for its effect on the human body, perceived by them as a hydraulic machine moved by the flow of juices.[39] Cornelis Bontekoe, one of the school's protagonists, thought eight to ten cups the minimum for one's health, but did not stop there. Rumoured to have been paid by the VOC to write favourably about the new drink, Bontekoe saw no problem with a daily intake of fifty to a hundred cups.[40]

Distilled liquor resembles tea in that it has retained the mystique of wholesomeness of a number of ailments, its demonization by many notwithstanding. Names such as aqua vitae, aquavit, and eau de vie illustrate its reputedly medicinal qualities. Well into the sixteenth century distillation remained within the alchemist tradition and was only practised by apothecaries. The above-mentioned Jean Liebault wrote one of the first descriptions of distilling in order to 'give apothecaries a taste of distilling and stimulate them to be more and more careful in preparing their medicines'.[41] The outcome of the process, brandy, was routinely used against diseases such as plague and gout and the loss of voice.[42] Late sixteenth-century Berlin restricted the sale of brandy to apothecaries,[43] while a generation later the French government even limited the privilege of manufacturing grain spirits to apothecaries and spice merchants.[44]

CONTROVERSY

It should scarcely be surprising that the introduction of the various exotic substances roused a great deal of debate in sixteenth- and seventeenth-century Europe. Nor is it strange that in the age of Reformation, Counter-Reformation, and Puritanism, these debates tended to be articulated in religious and moral terms, even if their true import was political or economic. The Reformation inaugurated a quest for personal salvation which centred on individual responsibility. Its ethic proclaimed salvation contingent upon self-restraint and discipline. Puritanism and its eighteenth-century successor movement, Pietism, laid even more stress on a practical morality for everyday life guided by sobriety and vigilance. The mind-altering effects of the various new stimulants alternatively fuelled fears of frivolousness and the spectre of a threatened moral order, or held out the promise of increased wakefulness, and as such inevitably figured in the deliberations of European clerics and moralists. A similar tone and substance is found in Russia, and the Islamic world, where the articulation of prohibitive measures as a 'return to the true faith' tended to be intertwined with efforts to bolster the legitimacy of (new) rulers.

Over time, debate in many countries subsided as the stimulants became irrelevant to medicine or lost their power as emblems of demonology. Even more deflecting was the shift in debate and opposition from moral preoccupation to economic concern. Moralists and preachers continued to inveigh against the satanic origin or the debilitating effect of tobacco, coffee, or liquor, but lost ground to bureaucrats who realized that the addictive substances, far from just draining bullion, might actually be turned into a source of profit. For the European early modern state, burdened by ever-growing military and administrative expenditure, tobacco, coffee, and liquor offered a welcome opportunity to expand its tax base.

With the exception of liquor, none of the stimulants became as frequent a target of official prohibition as tobacco. Rodrigo de Jerez, one of Columbus' crew and the first one to smoke in Europe, was brought before the Inquisition, accused of sorcery, and imprisoned for seven years upon his return to Spain.[45] In 1575 the colonial authorities in Mexico issued an order forbidding the use of tobacco throughout Spanish America. In some European countries, too, tobacco soon met a great obstacle in the abhorrence with which it was received by the authorities. In Elizabethan England, for instance, tobacco early on became the subject of fierce debate. Medical reservations, mercantilist concerns over the shortage of coin the importation of tobacco was thought to cause, as well as a deeply felt apprehension about the sloth and dissolution intemperance might produce among the working classes, caused many in the upper echelons of society to oppose the new 'drug'.[46] King James I, who received anti-tobacco counselling from his private surgeon, in 1604 took an active part in the debate and published a virulent attack on tobacco and its use, entitled *A Counterblast to Tobacco*, in which he elaborated on the prevailing association of tobacco with vanity and moral corruption. Tobacco, called repulsive in smell and dangerous for the brain by the king, was subjected to a tax, but not prohibited.

Charles I continued his father's policy of discouraging the use of tobacco, albeit less vigorously.[47] For both rulers, however, moral objections were balanced by a concern over the newly developed tobacco cultivation in America. At the behest of the Virginia tobacco lobby the crown in 1620 tried to limit the use of tobacco by banning cultivation in England. In 1627 this was followed by an attempt to regulate and centralize the importation of tobacco through an ordinance that required all tobacco coming into the country to go through London. This measure, which was renewed in 1630 and 1634, failed, as did the restriction of tobacco sales to licensed persons. Much as both James and Charles disliked tobacco, they gradually deferred to its economic benefits.

Economic considerations, not moral aversion, played a decisive role in the continuing discouragement of home-grown tobacco. Cromwell in 1652 bowed to the interests of the Virginia merchants by renewing the ban on indigenous cultivation. But the measure provoked so much resistance in Parliament that he was forced to mitigate the law to the point of non-enforcement. Thus all efforts to suppress cultivation and consumption ran aground against a habit which had become firmly rooted in social and economic life of the country and its colonies.

England was not unique with its royal opprobrium. In Denmark, too, the king personally objected to the smoking of tobacco. Simon Paulli, professor of botany and private physician of King Christian IV, wrote a treatise against tobacco at the ruler's instigation.[48] Elsewhere, the Church became the most vociferous opponent of tobacco. Pope

Urban VIII witnessed with growing concern how laymen and priests alike enjoyed their snuff even in church, and in 1642 issued a Bull against smoking in St Peter's, threatening violators with excommunication. Renewed by his successor Innocent X in 1650, the Bull was rendered ineffective by the granting, five years later, of a concession for the sale of tobacco and brandy in the papal domain. It was officially repealed by Pope Benedict XIII, who seems to have been an avid snuff taker himself.[49]

In Holland, where in medical circles tobacco roused the same curiosity as tea, doctors and public moralists differed in their opinion about its medicinal merits and its recreational permissibility.[50] While one Dutch doctor claimed that his smoking habit had helped him survive the plague of 1635–6,[51] a Flemish poet said that the 'two cordials' of the discovery of America, gold and tobacco, have 'done more mischief than the two great diseases, scurvy and the pocks'.[52] The most virulent vilification of smoking, or drinking tobacco, as it was called, came from the pulpit, even though opposition did not necessarily arise from clerical ranks. More typically, it was laymen who condemned smoking, associating it with vanity and idleness. None of this had much practical effect beyond the prohibition of tobacco in the Dutch navy and the land army of Prince Maurits.

The fire hazard, in addition to clerical resistance, led to a ban on smoking in many cities and principalities in German-speaking Europe after the peace of Westphalia. The city of Cologne issued a ban as early as 1649. Its example was followed three years later by Bavaria, which restricted prohibition to peasants and other commoners, by Saxony in 1653, and by Württemberg in 1656.[53] The city of Bern in 1661 outlawed the use of tobacco on the ground that it harmed human reproduction, and even instituted a tobacco court, which was only abolished in the mid-nineteenth century. In Austria tobacco was banned on a number of occasions in the late 1600s.[54] In some German towns restrictions on smoking in public remained in effect until the 1848 revolution.

Official aversion to tobacco, encouraged by the clergy, was not confined to western Europe. In Russia, a clerically-led reform movement persuaded Tsar Mikhail Romanov to prohibit the use of tobacco in 1634, promising deportation to Siberia for those who disobeyed him. Offenders risked being bastinadoed or having their nostrils slit – and at times the death penalty.[55] In 1649 Mikhail's successor Alexis, acting at the instigation of the puritanical 'Zealots of Piety', reaffirmed the ban in a new Law Code. The ban was enforced erratically and did little to stem the immense popularity of tobacco in Russia, but remained in place until 1697, when Peter the Great repealed it.

Further east, Shah 'Abbas of Iran (r. 1587–1629) outlawed the use of tobacco in the early 1600s, allegedly because it had been introduced by his archenemies, the Ottomans.[56] His successor, Shah Safi, repeated the ban when he acceded to the throne.[57] In the neighbouring Ottoman Empire, religious opinions were divided. Sultan Murad IV in 1633 used a huge fire that destroyed thousands of houses in Istanbul as a pretext to prohibit the use of a substance associated with political opposition.[58] The rulers of Japan and India outlawed tobacco as well in the early 1600s.[59] All this had little effect and, as in Russia and western Europe, tobacco smoking continued its unstoppable march in Asia.

Cocoa in Europe long remained a 'Catholic' drink prepared exclusively by Spanish monks in their cloisters. It met few adversaries, all of whom are found in the country's clerical circles. The main controversy over the use of chocolate in sixteenth-century Spain was whether it should be seen as a food or a liquid, with consequences for its use in periods of fasting in either case. Cocoa's alleged passion-raising properties also seem to have been a topic of discussion.[60]

In contrast to cocoa, tea in time became a quintessentially 'Calvinist' drink. Catholics and, to a lesser extent, Lutherans rarely treated alcohol as a major problem. Calvinism and Puritanism, on the other hand, tended to condemn alcohol as satanic and eagerly welcomed tea as an emblem of sobriety and moral restraint, almost as a divine alternative. England is a good example. There the incapacity of tea to intoxicate helped spur its acceptance in religious circles followed by social reformers concerned about the working classes. Even the Dutch physicians who described its effects in the bio-functional terms of their school – alcohol makes ill, tea heals – converged with more traditional religious views in crediting tea with increased vigilance and piousness.[61]

While tea by and large escaped the admonishments of seventeenth-century moralists, controversy was not altogether absent. An example of a written pronouncement against tea is the book by the above-mentioned Simon Paulli, which warns against the excessive use of tobacco as well as tea. The latter, the author notes, hastens the death of all past the age of forty.[62] In eighteenth-century England people like Jonas Hanway and John Wesley inveighed against tea for its allegedly effeminate aura and the indolence to which it was believed to lead.[63] Others reserved their invective for the 'superfluous money wasted on tea and sugar' by the poor.[64] In contemporary Germany, finally, the centralizing Prussian state campaigned against tea in the northern provinces it was bringing under its control, pronouncing the drink far less nutritious than the traditional beer in which it had an important economic stake.[65]

Coffee aroused far greater religious and political controversy when it
spread from the southern tip of the Arabian peninsula to other parts of
the Muslim world.[66] In the Ottoman Empire, religious leaders, who
watched in horror how the coffeehouse began to pose a challenge to the
mosque as a place of congregation, in the late sixteenth century
repeatedly urged the sultan to prohibit the use of coffee.[67] In Safavid
Iran, the scene of similar campaigns in 1645 and 1694, coffeehouses
rather than coffee were targeted.[68] While moral objections inspired the
ulama, secular authorities saw more cause for concern in the association
of coffeehouses with political debate. When during the Candia wars in
the 1660s tempers in coffeehouses ran high, the Ottoman Grand Vizier
Köprülü ordered their closure. The long-term official reception in the
Ottoman Empire was hardly less ambivalent than in Europe, however.
While religious aversion and a fear of social and political disruption led
to prohibitive measures, the income coffee generated eventually over-
came most resistance.[69]

The association of coffee with idleness and unrest was not confined to
the world of Islam. In Restoration England, too, coffee found opponents in those who saw in coffeehouses hotbeds of sedition and watched
their proliferation with suspicion. In an effort to muzzle the political
opinions voiced in the myriad new coffeehouses that sprang up after the
Great Fire of 1666, officials advised King Charles II to suppress these
'nurseries of idleness and pragmaticalness'. They received unexpected
assistance in their campaign from the women of London, who expressed
their concern about the side-effects of coffee drinking with the submission of a 'Women's Petition Against Coffee'. Calling coffee a beverage that caused domestic disorder and made men sexually inactive, the
women – who were not allowed in coffeehouses – complained that their
husbands spent idle time and money away from home, as a result of
which the 'entire race was in danger of extinction'.[70] These considerations eventually led the king to issue a proclamation in 1675, ordering
the closing of these establishments. Within ten days the measure had to
be repealed over a storm of popular protest.[71]

In most other European countries the introduction of coffee does not
seem to have been accompanied by much discussion beyond an occasional protest from wine purveyors or beer brewers who feared for their
livelihood. The only objection to coffee, François Valentyn wrote in the
early 1700s, came from suffering beer brewers.[72] Taxation rather than
prohibition became the norm in government reaction. The French
government, for instance, in 1692 monopolized coffee by instituting a
coffee tax and by restricting imports and sales to tax farmers. Taxation
motivated the English authorities as well. Seeing its revenue from beer

dwindle as coffee grew in popularity, the English government in 1663 was quick to license coffeehouses and levy an excise duty per gallon of coffee sold. As the enforcement of this tax was soon found to be rather cumbersome, it was replaced in 1689 by a simple customs duty of 5s per pound.

Germany was the exception to the rule of limited opposition to coffee. Resistance came in part from those who, wary of French influence, rejected coffee as a foreign drink and a fashionable luxury.[73] More serious was the mixture of state hunger for taxes and mercantilist fears of foreign imports, which made coffee fall under the axe of prohibitive measures for a good part of the eighteenth century. German officials assumed that large coffee imports would harm the sale of barley and malt used in the production of beer. The distinctly Prussian imprint of German attitudes toward coffee is reflected in the disciplinary character of official policy. Various German states in the eighteenth century issued decrees which forbade the consumption of coffee to the poor on the land and the working classes in the cities, allegedly in an effort to encourage public health but, more truthfully, in an attempt to protect the country's beer brewers. In some cases, ordinances that limited the enjoyment of coffee to nobles and clergymen led to popular revolt.[74] Abolitions of these and similar measures had to wait until the Napoleonic wars.

Given the visible effects on the immoderate user of alcohol, it is hardly surprising that the most adversarial reception of all was reserved for distilled liquor. From the Reformation onward, reactions in societies where Satan's abode, the tavern, was often found next door to the house of God tended to be expressed in stark moral language.[75] State measures meant to curb inebriation in seventeenth-century Europe were as numerous as clerical tirades against public intoxication: both are too numerous to list. However, just as government injunctions against spirits fought a losing battle against the need for tax revenue, so pious admonitions failed to deter the poor from indulging in their favourite vice.

Perhaps the best example is Russia, where the state began to monopolize the sale of alcohol as early as 1540. The profit-versus-morals dilemma was at the heart of the anti-liquor acts of 1649 and 1652. In part introduced at the behest of the church reform movement which encouraged people to attend church rather than spend time in taverns, in part to deflect precious grain from alcohol production, these acts curbed public drinking by abolishing the drink shops. The state, concerned about its tax revenue, simultaneously monopolized spirits, which yielded a higher tax profit than the traditional alcoholic beverages. The result of these prohibitionist measures was meagre, for illicit drinking places sprang up overnight. Naturally, state revenue fell drastically as well. In 1662 drink shops were reopened for the combined benefit of the thirsty population and the cash-hungry government.[76]

SPREAD AND POPULARIZATION

The substances examined here exhibit similarities not only in the patterns of their introduction and initial application but also in the manner in which they became disseminated and gained popularity among various segments of society.

As this process occurred in the context of the seventeenth-century commercial revolution, its near-simultaneity was anything but coincidental. Coffee, tea, and chocolate at first were exceedingly expensive drinks and therefore outside the reach of all but the well-to-do. As a regular supply system came into being, however, prices fell and the substances became more affordable.

But while the large-scale commercial traffic in new commodities accounts for their introduction and affordability, the explanation for their popular appeal cannot be reduced to mere availability. Other factors, relating to profound social changes that were simultaneously taking place in European society, merit consideration as well. Between 1500 and 1800, in the words of Roger Chartier, 'people [in the west] began to imagine, experience, and protect private life in a new way'.[77] Family life and individual freedom acquired new meanings as part of a redefinition of the boundaries between the public and private spheres. The encroachment of the bureaucratic state caused people to seek refuge in the intimacy of family life. At the same time, however, people sought to 'constitute a private life outside the constraints of the family', a private life, that is, on the basis of freely chosen forms of social and political association. The emerging administrative, commercial, and intellectual elites of Europe's secularizing urban centres engaged in new forms of social interaction, created new affiliations, and frequented new gathering places, ranging from Masonic Lodges to scientific societies and literary salons.

In this permutation of public and private spheres the stimulants played the role of tokens marking shifting class and gender lines. Except in the case of tobacco and liquor, popularization of what initially were expensive novelties occurred as a 'downward' movement, with ordinary people gradually adopting consumer habits that once were the exclusive domain of the wealthy who, in turn, often emulated the fashion of royal circles. In a desire to uphold class boundaries, society's upper strata tended to react to this by embracing a different stimulant or, eventually, by elevating the ambience of proper consumption to the level of exclusivity. No less salient in this process are the gender aspects. A clear differentiation between private and public space also became inscribed in a segregation between male and female spheres.

The popularization of tobacco followed a somewhat ambiguous trajectory in that the two opposite sides of the social spectrum acted as catalysts in its wider appeal. While sailors and soldiers spread tobacco among the common people, Europe's royal houses helped to popularize its use among the elite. An example is the transmission of the tobacco leaf from Lisbon to the French court, where the Queen Mother Catherine de Medici (r. 1560–89) developed a belief in its curative power. The adoption of the substance, which briefly came to be called *catherinaire*, precipitated its spread to other countries, where many were eager to imitate French ways. The sending of tobacco seeds to Italy by Cosimo de Medici's ambassador in Paris led to the cultivation of the plant in Tuscany. The papal nuntius in Lisbon simultaneously introduced the seeds to the Vatican, where they were planted in the gardens. Tobacco at this stage was associated with religious circles, as the name *herba santa* or *herba sacra* indicates.[78] The 'smoking sessions' various German courts organized in the early 1700s – the most renowned 'Tabak-Kollegium' being that of Frederick William of Prussia (1688– 1740) – accelerated the acceptance of tobacco among the elite beyond the Rhine.[79]

In the spread of tobacco we find perhaps the best example of a commodity whose varied use reflected social divisions. As tobacco smoke offended many in the upper classes and as pipe smoking was seen to be inelegant for ladies, taking snuff became a way for the elite to distinguish itself from the populace. Thus the Italian clergy mostly used tobacco in the form of snuff. Snuff was introduced in France under Louis XIII and became particularly popular at the court of Louis XIV, in part, it is said, because the king hated the smell of tobacco smoke.[80] From France the habit spread to other countries. England's upper classes adopted snuff under Charles II, who took to it while in Paris, and soon High Society shunned the pipe, which was relegated to the lower classes.[81] In Germany, finally, where snuff was introduced by French Huguenots after 1685, the manner in which social distinctions were marked by different ways of consuming tobacco is reflected in a satirical verse from the turn of the eighteenth century:

> Ein Landsknecht raucht, ein Höfling schnupft Tabak
> Doch wer ist hier am meisten fein?
> Der eine bläst ihn fort, der andre zieht ihn ein!

A mercenary smokes, a courtier snuffs tobacco
But who's the most refined here?
The one blows it out, the other inhales it![82]

Seventeenth-century Holland appears as something of an exception to this rule for, as Dutch genre painting suggests, pipe smoking was common among all classes. Scenes by painters such as Jan Steen and Adriaan Brouwer, while mostly depicting the labouring classes, show that in the United Provinces a wide range of social groups as well as both sexes enjoyed their pipes. With growing French influence in the eighteenth century, however, snuff became common among the upper ranks of Dutch society as well.

Unlike tobacco, which spread with lightning speed, coffee everywhere needed a few generations to become common. In the Ottoman Empire, where coffee had been known for a long time, popularization beyond Istanbul gained momentum in the late sixteenth and early seventeenth centuries, when coffeehouses opened in many provincial towns in Anatolia. In Europe, genuine popularization had to wait until the quandary between supply and demand had been solved. Maritime supply allowed for the quantities that made prices affordable and thus increased popularity. But only growing demand warranted increased supplies. In Holland, for instance, supplies did not reach substantial levels until the 1690s.[83]

Interestingly, Valentyn asserted that it was the English who had taught the Dutch to drink coffee.[84] Coffee indeed had been known somewhat longer in England, where it was introduced by Levantine merchants, who also opened the first coffeehouse in Oxford in 1650. London followed two years later. The drink quickly caught on, for a 1660 VOC report, commenting on an order for coffee from Amsterdam, noted that coffee was beginning to become popular in Europe, but 'especially in England'.[85] By 1661 London already boasted more than a dozen coffeehouses, a number which was to proliferate after the Great Fire of 1666.

Nevertheless, coffee deliveries from the east in these early days remained erratic, and the drink was therefore subject to great price fluctuations. It was only with the drop in prices in the early eighteenth century that coffee gained in popularity in England. Coffeehouses at that time began to spring up in the large cities and assumed an indispensable function as gathering places for those engaged in commerce and insurance. In Holland, meanwhile, where the first coffeehouse had been established in 1663–4,[86] there was 'hardly a house of standing where coffee is not drunk every morning'.[87] Not only people of standing, but even the 'little people', indeed the servants of the well-to-do, had acquired a taste for coffee.[88] Many coffeehouses in the larger Dutch cities were located in the vicinity of the stock exchange, where merchants and city administrators gathered to discuss and conduct business.

In France the court appears to have consumed coffee well before it was available to the general public. The country's first public coffee-house opened in 1672, but it had more success with newly introduced brandy than with coffee, which was little appreciated by the local population. This was to change with the opening of the famous coffee-house Procope in 1686. By distinguishing itself from the popular alcohol-purveying cabarets through a sumptuous decor and an air of sophistication, Procope managed to attract a high-class clientele that took advantage of the opportunity to gather separately from the common man. Soon others followed this example and coffeehouses proliferated.[89]

German-speaking Europe received its coffee not just from the west but, bordering as it did on Ottoman territory, acquired it via the eastern overland trade as well. Vienna, Regensburg, and Nuremberg came into contact with coffee through the Turks. Vienna had four coffeehouses in 1688, a number that was to grow to sixty-eight in 1787.[90] Due to their proximity to Holland, the western regions tended to receive their supply via the East India trade. Just as the English taught the Dutch to drink coffee, the latter spread the drink to Germany. Coffee was introduced at the court of Brandenburg by the above-mentioned Bontekoe, who was the private physician of Frederick William. The acceptance at the elite level must have stimulated con-sumption in coffeehouses, the first of which was opened in 1671 in Hamburg. Often established and run by foreigners, coffeehouses soon spread to other places as well.[91] Yet in Germany, too, where coffee-houses lacked the Dutch and English association with commercial vitality, coffee long remained an exclusive drink and, as elsewhere, the middle classes only took to it in the early eighteenth century. At that time special coffee sessions, so-called 'Kaffeekränzchen', began to be organized by and for women. These gatherings were occasions for the exchange of news and gossip, and may be seen as the female response to the coffeehouses which by then had clearly become a male domain.

The story of the popularization of chocolate runs somewhat parallel to that of coffee. Due to a lack of familiarity with cacao following Spanish secrecy, the Dutch or the English in the sixteenth century would take all they deemed valuable upon capturing a Spanish ship but throw overboard any cacao they found.[92] By the beginning of the next century, however, word of the new drink began to spread. Italy was the first country after Spain that became familiar with cocoa. In 1606 the drink was known in Florence. The breakthrough north of the Pyrenees came in 1615, when Anna of Austria, the eldest child of King Philip III, was married to Louis XIII and offered Spanish chocolate to her new husband as part of her bridal gift. The drink rapidly gained ground among French courtiers, its popularity helped by the status of Spain as the origin of fashionable and chic trends.

Following Spain, France quickly imbued cocoa with an aura of sensuality and luxury. Louis XIV and his Spanish wife Maria Theresa continued the court's infatuation with chocolate. Soon France made itself more independent from Spanish supplies by cultivating cacao beans in its own West Indian colonies. The aftermath of the War of the Spanish Succession also brought cocoa to the Austrian domains of Spain where, due to low taxation, it became a popular drink among the aristocracy and the wealthy.

Holland and England became active in the transshipment of cacao – Amsterdam became the largest port of entry following the Dutch seizure of Curaçao in 1634 – but consumption in both countries seems to have been introduced from France. In Amsterdam various coffee-houses offered chocolate around 1665.[93] In London's early coffee-houses chocolate was still served as a cold drink – eating chocolate only began in the nineteenth century with the invention of a method to combine cocoa butter with chocolate liquor. In 1657 a Parisian shop-keeper established the first chocolate shop in the English capital. The price in the mid-seventeenth century of 10s to 15s per pound made chocolate, even more than coffee, an exclusive beverage, a status it retained throughout the eighteenth century. A few of London's early chocolate houses, such as White's Cocoa House, later turned into respectable clubs for the aristocracy.

As well as in its East Asian lands of origin, tea established itself as the favourite drink primarily in the north-west European countries active in importing it. Otherwise, tea became a household beverage in those countries and regions where religious reform movements were most keen to propagate an alternative to alcohol. These include, besides Holland and England, the United States, at least until 1773, most of northern Germany, and Russia, where tea became a national drink as well, albeit not until the end of the eighteenth century. Exceptions to this pattern are the countries in south-west and south Asia, from Turkey to India, which also adopted tea. There, changing trade routes, the feasibility of indigenous cultivation, and the growing influence of Britain, British India, and, in the case of Turkey and Iran, Russia, caused tea to replace coffee in the nineteenth century.

As was noted before, England initially received its tea via Holland. The first direct delivery from China to England seems to have taken place in 1666, four years after the coming of Catherine of Braganza from Portugal as Charles II's bride had introduced tea as a fashionable drink for ladies.[94] For some time to come, however, tea continued to be considered 'a rarity' and lagged behind coffee in popularity.[95]

The main reason for this was that tea, more than coffee, was prohibitively expensive at 60s a pound or eight times the weekly wages of a labourer. As long as the supply was dependent on private merchants, tea deliveries remained scanty and erratic. This situation ended when in 1686 the EIC decided to include tea in its regular imports from Asia. The result was a great increase in the quantities supplied. Whereas less than 200 pounds had annually been delivered in most of the period from 1675 to 1686, almost 5,000 pounds was imported in 1687, while three years later the company shipped over 40,000 pounds.[96] In the process the EIC gained the upper hand over the private traders who dominated the coffee trade.

A good example of shifting consumer habits is eighteenth-century England, which saw the decline of the coffeehouse and the rise of the tea garden, catering to men, women, and families.[97] Curiously, tea in the course of time became Britain's democratic drink par excellence. The beginning of tea's downward movement was facilitated by its noted reputation as a drink without intoxicating properties. Unlike coffee, which was rumoured to be 'bad for the head', tea was also recommended for ladies as much as for gentlemen. An influential periodical such as the *Spectator* in the early eighteenth century no doubt further contributed to this when it advised its readers that 'all well-regulated households served tea in the morning'.[98]

Even so, the tax slapped on it by the English government – instituted in tandem with that on coffee – long continued to make tea unattainable for the masses. A flourishing black market was the result. Large-scale smuggling did not stop until 1784 when William Pitt repealed the high government duties and caused the EIC to import enough tea to satisfy demand without raising prices. Tea by then was no longer seen as an exclusively upper-class beverage: originally consumed unsweetened, it was now taken with sugar – now affordable as well – and had become the indispensable drink for the English working classes starved for cheap calories.[99]

Protestant Holland, as England, did not really become a tea-drinking country until the turn of the eighteenth century. Doctor Bontekoe's approval may have had some influence on popular acceptance, but falling prices, resulting from regular supplies, are likely to have played a greater role. The growing popularity of tea in Holland in the early eighteenth century is illustrated in the increasing amounts shipped by the VOC. In 1691 the Amsterdam directors of the company, no doubt encouraged by the recent English decision to allow the import of tea from Holland by licence, issued an order for 15,000 to 20,000 pounds.[100] In 1715, 60,000 to 70,000 pounds were requested for the home country; in the following year the order went up to 100,000 pounds, reaching 1 million pounds in 1724.[101]

Beer and ale for centuries had provided nutrition for the labouring classes in northern countries. Judging from the description various travellers gave of public drunkenness of men and women in the early 1600s, distilled liquor may have replaced these drinks in Russia earlier than in western Europe.[102] There, spirits continued to be used medicinally until the mid- and late seventeenth century, when brandy began to be consumed in some quantity.[103] Brandy consumption received a fillip when in European armies it became customary for soldiers to drink before engaging in battle. Indeed, some hold the land wars of the late seventeenth century and in particular the campaign waged by Louis XIV against Holland in 1672 responsible for the spreading popularity of spirits.[104]

Nor did grain-based spirits become popular in north-western Europe before the mid-seventeenth century. Changes in technology had some impact on this development, for large-scale distilling became possible only with the improvement of distilling apparatus. Cheap and easy access to ingredients played a role as well. Baltic grain, entering Holland in unprecedented quantities, came to be used for the manufacture of Dutch gin or genever. The distilleries that sprang up in the town of Schiedam around 1630 profited from these cheap imports as well as from the fact that distillers learned how to make their own yeast.[105] The lower price of grain-based liquors compared to wine or sugar-based ones such as rum contributed to a quick spread among various social classes. As a result, the number of distilleries in Schiedam increased from 11 in 1650 to 120 in 1775.[106]

The availability of cheap sugar similarly reduced the cost of manufacturing sugar-based spirits.[107] This development continued thanks to the establishment of a West Indian sugar economy. Rum, made from sugar cane, was popularized following the capture of Jamaica in 1655. It replaced beer in the British navy. True popularity, however, remained confined to England and Holland, the countries whose West India Companies imported most of it from overseas.

Introduced in the seventeenth century, liquor followed the other substances in gaining a solid place in people's diets in the eighteenth century. In England, for instance, gin began to rank with beer and ale as the favourite drink of the labouring classes in part as a result of a government promotion of indigenous spirits. The quantity of British spirits on which duty was charged increased from about 800,000 gallons in 1694 to over 6,000,000 in 1736.[108] So popular did gin become among the masses that anxiety about the state of productivity and public morality led to a reversal in state policy in the form of the prohibitionist Gin Act. The Act came too late to be effective, however. By the time it was passed, liquor had become too much of a popular drink to be curtailed. Not even tea, the alternative espoused by social reformers, was able to accomplish that feat.

CONCLUSION

The seventeenth and early eighteenth centuries witnessed the rapid global spread of tobacco, coffee, cocoa, tea, and distilled spirits. With the exception of liquor, all were introduced from newly discovered lands and therefore held out the promise as much as the threat of the unknown. Heralded for their medicinal qualities by some, they were greeted with suspicion by others. Doctors, pursuing new avenues of medical insight, debated the wholesome qualities of coffee and cocoa, claiming them to be alternatively beneficial or detrimental to the body and the mind. Everywhere preachers railed against the supposedly diabolical properties of tobacco and liquor.

If discoveries, missionaries, and adventurers were responsible for the acquaintance with the stimulants, private merchants, sailors, and soldiers further disseminated them around the globe. Levantine traders were instrumental in the spread of coffee; soldiers brought cocoa and tobacco with them across the Pyrenees. At the other end of the social spectrum, European royals, embracing chocolate and tea, stimulated and accelerated their adoption by elites.

Introduced in a period of worldwide religious ferment, the substances evoked apprehensions that resonated with the social transformation introduced by Protestantism in the west and the appropriation of religious symbols in the bureaucratic empires of Islam. Prescribing discipline and sobriety, European reform movements stressed individual responsibility as a prerequisite for salvation, and evaluated the stimulants on the degree to which they accorded with a life of moral restraint and moderation. A secularized variant, especially active in eighteenth-century Britain and Germany, demonized those stimulants it saw as undermining the moral fibre of the poor.

Fierce controversy notwithstanding, the quantities consumed in the first half century of introduction were without exception small. Supply, accordingly, was intermittent and weakly organized. This situation only changed when the newly established East and West India Companies began to include the commodities in their commercial activities. Sustained deliveries ensured guaranteed supplies, which in turn brought down prices to levels that made consumption affordable beyond the wealthy. A mass market, however, came into being only in the eighteenth century, when the stimulants had trickled down to the labouring classes for whom they provided the sole relief in a dreary life and a necessary dietary component.

The state everywhere played an important role in this latter process. At first wary of, or indifferent to, the new commodities, it quickly realized the potential profits accruing from mass consumption. The persistence of religious or moral sentiments that favoured curbing measures notwithstanding, bans were never enforced for long and, before long, revenue-hungry governments even began to stimulate consumption. The duties they imposed caused prices to go up, but the legalization and orderly distribution that accompanied taxation also spurred further growth in trade and consumption.

Neither increased availability at affordable prices nor mere state encouragement could have brought about the rising popularity of the stimulants at the turn of the eighteenth century. Religious and social moralism contributed to increased consumption by welcoming those stimulants whose intoxicating qualities were negligible. The main catalyst, however, was a changing social climate in western Europe, embodied by a burgeoning entrepreneurial class, prospering on new commercial and financial opportunities and open to new products brought from afar. Tobacco, coffee, chocolate, and tea gained widespread popularity in the contexts of the rise of new forms of entertainment, new forms of assembly, and new affiliations. Coffeehouses, salons, lodges, and clubs emerged as new venues for the expanding urban citizenry or simply for men who sought to escape the confinement of their homes.

In this development both class and gender differences became inscribed in the nature of the stimulants and the places where they thrived. Taverns, once the gathering place for a variegated crowd, now turned into the precinct of the labouring classes, their role as centres of culture and entertainment for respectable citizens taken over by coffeehouses. The latter, in turn, over time lost their preeminence to the private club, where commoners had no place. Whereas an incipient bourgeoisie, endowed with increasing financial means and an appetite for the exotic, embraced snuff, developed a taste for coffee, and consumed chocolate in elegant surroundings, the labouring classes began to frequent taverns and drink shops where tobacco and spirits provided oblivion. The business men began to conduct in coffeehouses, finally, relegated women to the exchange of gossip over coffee and tea in the private sphere.

ACKNOWLEDGEMENTS

I would like to thank Professor Nikki Keddie for drawing my attention to the remarkable similarities between the spread of the various substances discussed here and for encouraging me to write this essay.

NOTES

1 Strictly speaking, sugar should be considered in this category as well, especially since it bears a striking resemblance to the substances discussed in this essay in the way it was perceived in sixteenth- to eighteenth-century Europe. I have chosen not to include sugar, however, because for most of the period considered here sugar was seen and used as a spice, and as an ancillary substance rather than a separate stimulant. For sugar, the reader is referred to Sidney W. Mintz, *Sweetness and Power: The Place of Sugar in Modern History* (New York, 1985). Its title notwithstanding, this otherwise excellent book focuses primarily on the Anglo-Saxon world in its discussion of the spread of sugar.

2 Some have claimed that tobacco originated in Africa and was used in various parts of the world prior to its introduction in Europe. See, for example, Leo Wiener, *Africa and the Discovery of America*, 3 vols. (Philadelphia, 1920–2), I; and Lotherd Becker, 'Zur Ethnologie der Tabakspfeife', in Sergius Golowin, ed., *Kult und Brauch der Kräuterpfeife in Europa* (Allmendingen, 1982), pp. 5–25. For a refutation of the non-American origin of tobacco, see Günther Stahl, 'Zur Frage des Ursprungs des Tabaksrauchens', *Anthropos*, 26 (1931), pp. 569–82. The use of tobacco in South America is exhaustively discussed by Johannes Wilbert, *Tobacco and Shamanism in South America* (New Haven, 1987).

3 G. A. Brongers, *Pijpen en tabak* (Bussum, 1964), p. 14; Ned Rival, *Tabac, miroir du temps* (Paris, 1982), p. 13.

4 See Jacob M. Price, 'The Tobacco Adventure to Russia: Enterprise, Politics, and Diplomacy in the Quest for a Northern Market for English Colonial Tobacco, 1676–1722', *Transactions of the American Philosophical Society*, n.s., 51 (1961), p. 8.

5 G. D. J. Schotel, *Letterkundige bijdragen tot de geschiedenis van den tabak, de koffij en de thee* (The Hague, 1848), p. 81; Friedrich Tiedemann, *Geschichte des Tabaks und anderer ähnlicher Genussmittel* (Frankfurt a/M, 1854), pp. 165–6.

6 Tiedemann, *Geschichte des Tabaks*, p. 191.

7 See Ernest M. Satow, 'The Introduction of Tobacco into Japan', *Transactions of the Asiatic Society of Japan*, 6 (1878), pp. 68–84.

8 This information is derived from Gillian Wagner, *The Chocolate Conscience* (London, 1987), pp. 7–18.

9 See Robert J. Ferry, *The Colonial Elite of Early Caracas: Formation and Crisis 1567–1767* (Berkeley, 1989), pp. 45ff.

10 For coffee in the Ottoman Empire, see Ralph S. Hattox, *Coffee and Coffeehouses: The Origins of a Social Beverage in the Medieval Near East* (Seattle, 1985).

11 See Don Garcia de Silva y Figueroa, *Comentarios de D. Garcia y Figueroa de la embajada que del parte del Rey de Espana Don Felipe III hize al Rey Xa Abas de Persia*, 2 vols. (Madrid, 1903), II, pp. 378–83; and Pietro della Valle, *Viaggi di Pietro della Valle*, 2 vols. (Brighton, 1843), II, p. 25; and Fedot Kotov, *Khozhenie kuptsa Kotova v Persiyu*, ed. N. A. Kutznetsova (Moscow, 1958), pp. 43, 80–1. See also Rudi Matthee, 'Coffee in Safavid Iran: Commerce and Consumption', *Journal of the Economic and Social History of the Orient*, 37 (1994), pp. 1–32.

12 Leonhard Rauwolf, *Aigentliche Beschreibung der Raiss . . . inn die Morgenländer* (Laugingen, 1582; repr. Graz, 1971), pp. 102–3.

13 In Prosper Alpinus, *De plantis Aegypti liber* (Venice, 1592), p. 62.

14 See W. Ph. Coolhaas, ed., *Pieter van den Broecke in Azië*, 2 vols. (The Hague, 1962), I, pp. 92 and 107.

15 For the early Dutch coffee trade from Mokha, see C. G. Brouwer, *Cauwa ende Comptanten: De Verenigde Oostindische Compagnie in Jemen 1614–1655/The Dutch East India Company in Yemen 1614–1655* (Amsterdam, 1988).

16 W. Ph. Coolhaas, ed., *Generale Missiven van Gouverneurs-Generaal en Raden aan Heren XVII der Verenigde Oostindische Compagnie*, vol. II: *1639–1655* (The Hague, 1964), p. 114; and J. A. van Chijs, ed. *Dagh-Register gehouden int Casteel Batavia Anno 1661* (Batavia and The Hague, 1890), p. 3.

17 William H. Ukers, *The Romance of Tea: An Outline History of Tea and Tea-Drinking through Sixteen Hundred Years* (New York, 1936), pp. 52–5.

18 T. Volker, *Porcelain and the Dutch East India Company* (Leiden, 1954), p. 48.

19 See Sir Henry Yule, *Hobson-Jobson* (London, 1886; repr. 1985), p. 906.

20 See John Bruce, *Annals of the Honorable East-India Company*, 3 vols. (London, 1810; repr. 1986), II, 210–11.

21 John J. McCusker, 'Distilling and its Implications for the Atlantic World of the Seventeenth and Eighteenth Centuries', in *Production, Marketing and Consumption of Alcoholic Beverages since the Late Middle Ages, Proceedings Tenth International Economic History Congress* (Louvain, 1990), pp. 7–19.

22 R. E. F. Smith and David Christian, *Bread and Salt: A Social and Economic History of Food and Drink in Russia* (Cambridge, 1984), p. 89.

23 Vera Efron, 'The Tavern and Saloon in Old Russia', *Quarterly Journal of Studies on Alcohol*, 16 (1955), p. 494.

24 Rival, *Tabac*, p. 12.

25 See Brongers, *Pijpen*, pp. 16–25.

26 Count Corti, *A History of Smoking*, trans. from German by Paul England (London, n.d.), pp. 99–100, 167.

27 Rival, *Tabac*, p. 15; C. M. MacInnes, *The Early English Tobacco Trade* (London, 1926), pp. 16–16; Simon Schama, *The Embarrassment of Riches: An Interpretation of Dutch Culture in the Golden Age* (New York, 1987), p. 197.

28 P. K. Gode, 'References to Tobacco in some Sanskrit Works between AD 1600 and 1900', *Studies in Indian Cultural History*, 1 (Hoshiarpur, 1961), p. 415.

29 Wolfgang Schivelbusch, *Das Paradies, der Geschmack und die Vernunft: Eine Geschichte der Genussmittel* (Munich, 1980), p. 99.

30 Henry Stubbe (Stubbs), *The Indian Nectar or Discourse concerning Chocolata* (London, 1662), p. 35.

31 Thomas Herbert, *Some Years Travel into Divers Parts of Africa, and Asia the Great* (London, 1638), p. 241.

32 Philippe Sylvestre Dufour, *Traitez nouveaux et curieux du café, du thé et du chocolate* (The Hague, 1685), pp. 113–16.

33 Algemeen Rijks Archief (Dutch National Archives, The Hague), *Verenigde Oostindische Compagnie* (VOC) 1185, 29 Aug. 1650, fol. 618.

34 Aytoun Ellis, *The Penny Universities: A History of the Coffee-Houses* (London, 1956), p. 15.

35 For the early Arabic manuals, see Hattox, *Coffee and Coffeehouses*, pp. 61–71. Examples of Persian botanical dictionaries are Muhammad Mu'min Husayni, *Tuhfah-i Hakim Mu'min* (Tehran, n.d.; new edn, 1360/1981–2), p. 212; new edn, p. 697; and the ones discussed in K. Seligmann, *Ueber drey höchst seltene persische Handschriften: Ein Beitrag zur Litteratur der orientalischen Arzneymittellehre* (Vienna, 1833); and Aladin Goushegir, 'Le café en Iran des Safavides aux Qajar à l'époque actuelle', in Hélène Desmet-Grégoire, ed., *Contributions au thème du et des cafés dans les sociétés du Proche-Orient* (Aix-en-Provence, 1991), pp. 75–112.

36 Ellis, *Penny Universities*, p. 74.

37 Ukers, *Romance of Tea*, pp. 66–7.

38 Smith and Christian, *Bread and Salt*, p. 230.

39 Karl Wassenberg, *Tee in Ostfriesland: vom religiösen Wundertrank zum profanen Volksgetränk* (Leer, 1991), pp. 67–94.

40 Schama, *Embarrassment*, p. 172. Bontekoe was certainly handsomely rewarded by the East India Company *after* he had written his book.

41 Gregory A. Austin, *Alcohol in Western Society from Antiquity to 1800* (Santa Barbara, Calif., 1985), p. 176.

42 Fernand Braudel, *Capitalism and Material Life, 1400–1800*, English trans. Siyân Reynolds (London, 1973), p. 171.

43 Austin, *Alcohol*, p. 178.

44 *Ibid.*, p. 218.

45 Corti, *History of Smoking*, pp. 38–9, 50; Rival, *Tabac*, p. 13.

46 Larry Harrison, 'Tobacco Battered and the Pipes Shattered: A Note on the Fate of the First British Campaign against Tobacco Smoking', *British Journal of Addiction*, 81 (1986), pp. 553–8.

47 MacInnes, *Early English Tobacco Trade*, p. 82.

48 D. Simonis Paulli, *Commentarius de abusu tabaci et herbae thée* (n.p., 1665).

49 Tiedemann, *Geschichte des Tabaks*, pp. 143–4; Corti, *History of Smoking*, pp. 128–32, 198–9.

50 Brongers, *Pijpen*, p. 37. See also John Landwehr, *De Nederlander uit en thuis: Spiegel van het dagelijkse leven uit bijzondere zeventiende-eeuwse boeken* (Alphen a/d Rijn, 1981), pp. 63–5.

51 Schama, *Embarrassment*, p. 197.

52 In the anonymous 'Tobacco Battered and the Pipes Shattered, Collected out of the Famous Poems of Joshua Sylvester, Gent', which, in turn, is included in the anonymous *The Touchstone or Trial of Tobacco . . . with a Word of Advice against Immoderate Drinking and Smoaking* (London, 1676). James I's *A Counterblast to Tobacco* is included as well.

53 Corti, *History of Smoking*, pp. 109–16.

54 *Ibid.*, pp. 166–8.

55 Adam Olearius, *Vermehrte newe Beschreibung der Muscowitischen und Persischen Reyse* (Schleswig, 1656; repr. Tübingen, 1971), pp. 197, 269, 273–4.

56 *Ibid.*, p. 645.

57 Abu'l Hasan Qazvini, *Fawa'id al-Safawiyah*, ed. Miryam Mir Ahmadi (Tehran, 1367/1988–9), p. 48; and Jean-Baptiste Tavernier, *Les six voyages de Jean Bapt. Tavernier en Turquie, en Perse, et aux Indes*, 2 vols. (Utrecht, 1712), I, p. 599.

58 Hans Joachim Kissling, 'Zur Geschichte der Rausch- und Genussgifte im Osmanischen Reiche', *Südostforschungen*, 16 (1957), pp. 346–7.

59 P. K. Gode, 'The History of Tobacco in India and Europe between AD 1500 and 1800', *Studies in Indian Cultural History*, I (Hoshiarpur, 1961), pp. 431–2.

60 Wagner, *Chocolate Conscience*, p. 10; Brandon Head, *The Food of the Gods: A Popular Account of Chocolate* (London, n.d.), p. 79. For bibliographical references, see Schotel, *Letterkundige bijdragen*, p. 143.

61 Wassenberg, *Tee in Ostfriesland*, pp. 84–6.

62 Paulli, *Commentarius*.

63 Ukers, *Romance of Tea*, pp. 80–2.

64 Words of Arthur Young, quoted in Gervas Huxley, *Talking of Tea* (London, 1956), p. 10.

65 Wassenberg, *Tee in Ostfriesland*, pp. 106–13.

66 See Hattox, *Coffee and Coffeehouses*, pp. 29ff.

67 See François Valentyn, *Oost en Nieuw Oost-Indiën*, 5 vols. (Dordrecht and Amsterdam, 1726), V, 194–5.

68 For anti-coffeehouse measures in Safavid Iran, see Matthee, 'Coffee in Safavid Iran'.

69 Suraiya Faroqhi, 'Coffee and Spices: Official Ottoman Reactions to Egyptian Trade in the Later Sixteenth Century', Festschrift für Andreas Tietze, *Wiener Zeitschrift für die Kunde des Morgenlandes*, 76 (1986), pp. 89–93.

70 W. Ukers, *All about Coffee* (New York, 1935), pp. 66–7; and Ellis, *Penny-Universities*, p. 88.

71 Ellis, *Penny Universities*, pp. 94–7.

72 Valentyn, *Oost-Indiën*, V, p. 198.

73 Ulla Heise, *Coffee and Coffee Houses*, transl. from German (West Chester, Pa., 1987), pp. 37–9.

74 *Ibid.*, pp. 38–8.

75 Th. van Deursen, *Het kopergeld van de Gouden Eeuw*, vol. II: *Volkskultuur* (Assen and Amsterdam, 1978), p. 38.

76 Smith and Christian, *Bread and Salt*, pp. 151ff.

77 Philippe Ariès and George Duby, eds., *A History of Private Life*, vol. III: *Passions of the Renaissance* (Cambridge, Mass., 1989), p. 399.

78 Rival, *Tabac*, pp. 18–20; Corti, *History of Smoking*, pp. 58–60, 63–4.

79 Werne Kloos, *Tabak-Kollegium: Ein Kulturgeschichtlicher Almanach für den Raucher* (Bremen, 1967), p. 31.

80 *Ibid.*, pp. 80–1.

81 Corti, *History of Smoking*, pp. 187–8.

82 Quoted in *ibid.*, p. 26.

83 Kristoff Glamann, *Dutch-Asiatic Trade, 1620–1740* (Copenhagen and The Hague, 1958), p. 183.

84 Valentijn, *Oost-Indiën*, v, p. 190.

85 Coolhaas, *Generale Missiven*, vol. III: *1655–1674* (1968), p. 310.

86 See Dick Adelaar, '"Turkse" genotmiddelen in Nederland: koffie en tabak', Hans Theunissen *et al.*, eds., *Topkapi & Turkomanie: Turks-Nederlandse ontmoetingen sinds 1600* (Amsterdam, 1989), p. 159.

87 Valentyn, *Oost-Indiën*, v, p. 190.

88 *Ibid.*

89 See Thomas Brennan, *Public Drinking and Popular Culture in Eighteenth-Century Paris* (Princeton, 1988), pp. 85, 132; Schotel, *Letterkundige bijdragen*, pp. 138–9.

90 See Günther Schiedlausky, *Tee, Kaffee, Schokolade* (Munich, 1961), pp. 15–16.

91 *Ibid.*, p. 166.

92 Marcia and Frederic Morton, *Chocolate: An Illustrated History* (New York, 1986), pp. 11–12.

93 J. Feenstra, 'Wacht U voor koffiepraat: De eerste koffiehuizen in Amsterdam en hun ontwikkeling', *Ons Amsterdam*, 14:4 (1962), p. 106.

94 Ukers, *Romance of Tea*, pp. 76–7.

95 W. Milburn, *Oriental Commerce*, 2 vols. (London, 1813), II, p. 531.

96 These figures are given in *ibid.*, II, pp. 531–2.

97 Huxley, *Talking of Tea*, p. 79.

98 Quoted in Agnes Repplier, *To Think of Tea!* (Boston and New York, 1932), p. 33.

99 For this, see Mintz, *Sweetness and Power*.

100 Coolhaas, *Generale Missiven*, vol. V: *1686–1697* (1975), p. 407.

101 *Ibid.*, pp. 220–1.

102 See Boris M. Segal, *Russian Drinking: Use and Abuse of Alcohol in Pre-Revolutionary Russia* (New Brunswick, 1987), pp. 31–6.

103 Austin, *Alcohol*, p. 250.

104 *Ibid.*, p. 264.

105 *Ibid.*, pp. 178, 183, 205.

106 Schama, *Embarrassment*, p. 193.

107 See McCusker, 'Distilling and its Implications'.

108 James Samuelson, *The History of Drink: A Review, Social, Scientific, and Political* (London, 1878), pp. 160–1.

injection.[13] Having injected a warm solution of opium into the crural vein of a dog, Christopher Wren (1632–1723) and Robert Boyle (1627–91) noted that the animal appeared extremely 'stupified'.[14] In animal experiments of the same kind, Johann Daniel Major (1634–93) and Johann Sigismund Elsholtz (1623–88) induced drowsiness and sleep with opium injections. Elsholtz particularly convinced himself of the narcotic and analgesic effects of the drug: since his experimental animal was a hound, he tried to wake it up by shouting hunting commands, and occasionally he pricked the sleeping dog's tongue or one of its legs with a needle.[15] It must be emphasized, however, that these early injection experiments were *not* specifically directed towards a study of the pharmacology of opium. The main concern was the new method of application, and the significance of the observed experimental effects consisted in the mere fact that they were basically the same as those following oral administration (which were known from medical practice).

Other early experiments dealt with the acute toxicity of opium. In 1678/9 William Courten (1642–1702) studied the effects of several vegetable, animal, and mineral poisons in dogs and other warm-blooded animals. Again deep sleep was the characteristic symptom following both peroral and intravenous giving of opium. After intravenous injection, however, the effects appeared more rapidly, included violent convulsions, and ultimately led to death. Courten administered very high doses, ranging from 50 to 120 grains.[16] (The usual therapeutic dose in human beings was one or two grains of opium.[17]) Occasionally he carried out post-mortem examinations of his poisoned animals. Yet in opening a cat, which had been killed by intravenous injection of opium, he only remarked that he 'did not find the Blood much altered from its Natural State'.[18] Courten did not use his observations to formulate any theory on the mode of action of the drug. It seems that he was merely interested in producing and describing characteristic symptoms of intoxications.

Courten's experiments were published only in 1712, ten years after his death, when Hans Sloane (1660–1753) communicated an English translation of the original Latin manuscript to the Royal Society. In the preceding decade, however, some experiments with opium had been made which were already connected with theoretical considerations on its mode of action. The aforementioned early eighteenth-century theory that the observable effects of opiates resulted from rarefaction of the blood was for the most part an iatromechanical speculation. Stupor and sleep, for example, were explained as following from a compression of the nervous tubuli or fibres in the brain by turgid cerebral vessels, which were distended by the thinned blood.[19] Yet, some early advocates of this theory, such as Richard Mead (1673–1754), John Freind (1675–1728), and the Wittenberg medical professor Johann Gottfried Berger (1659–1736), tried to produce some experimental evidence as well: their dissections of dogs and cats which had been killed by orally or intravenously administered solutions of opium showed that the blood vessels were actually turgid and that the blood was thin. Berger also opened the skulls of living dogs, which were somnolent and stupefied from opium, and found the same. Freind made additional *in vitro* experiments with freshly extracted arterial blood of a dog and with human serum. Admixing the Liquid Panacea of Dr Jones (i.e. a water solution of opium) and Sydenham's Laudanum liquidum (i.e. a solution of opium in Spanish wine), he noted that the blood and the serum became thinner in both trials and that the blood kept its shining red colour.[20] Still it would be wrong to assume that the quoted authors actually *founded* their 'rarefaction theory' (as it might be called) on pharmacological experimentation. They used their experimental findings merely as one of several 'arguments' (as Freind put it) in favour of the theory, and they attributed the same epistemological status to their highly speculative interpretations of the known clinical effects and of certain chemical properties of the drug.[21]

EXPERIMENTAL STUDIES

Actual pharmacological research on opium did not start before 1742, when Charles Alston (1683–1760), Professor of Botany and Materia Medica at the University of Edinburgh, published a number of experiments within a general dissertation on the drug. Alston combined the hitherto employed experimental methods and enlarged their spectrum: he administered opium to animals orally, intravenously, and externally, using dogs and frogs; like Freind he made *in vitro* trials; and he experimented on himself. More importantly, he put current views on opium to the experimental test.[22]

With respect to the 'rarefaction theory' Alston microscopically studied the blood flow in the capillaries of the webbed feet of frogs, which had been given orally a water solution of opium: the blood changed neither its consistency nor its colour, yet the flow significantly slowed down. Mixing *in vitro* the water solution as well as Sydenham's Laudanum with freshly let blood he observed rather coagulation and precipitation than rarefaction. Accordingly, Alston disagreed with the theory of rarefied blood.[23] His self-experimentation referred to the current practice of applying opium externally to painful areas. Opium plasters applied to his little finger and his arm for a whole night did not produce any effect at all, and a solution of opium in water poured on excoriated parts and in superficial wounds caused burning pain. '*Opium* is not', he concluded, 'properly speaking, narcotick externally; and there may be Pains which it cannot remove as a Topick'.[24]

Alston's experiments foreshadowed the different directions of pharmacological research on opium that were to be pursued in the next fifty years or so. A large part of experimentation aimed at finding out the real mode of action of the drug.[25] A second area of scientific interest was the effects of opium on heart activity and blood circulation. And thirdly, experiments were carried out in order to answer certain questions of current opium therapy.

Exploring the basic mode of action

Alston's own theory of the way opiates primarily acted on the body was derived more from clinical experience than from experimental work. For instance, he pointed out that in cases of violent tenesmus the intake of a few drops of Laudanum liquidum almost immediately eased the pain, and that it stopped vomiting 'almost as soon'. This meant – in his opinion – that the remedy acted long before it could have been absorbed and conveyed in the blood. That is why Alston concluded that opium affected 'first and principally' the nerves of the parts to which it was applied, i.e. in case of oral taking, the extremities of nerves in the walls of the stomach. These peripheral impressions would then be quickly distributed 'by Consent' or by sympathy through the whole nervous system.[26] This was basically not a new theory, since the Swiss physician Johann Jakob Wepfer (1620–95), the seventeenth-century authority in the field of toxicology, had already taken a very similar view in the late 1670s.[27] Dissecting or vivisecting perorally poisoned animals, the latter had observed that some drugs caused grave symptoms, though they had apparently not yet left the stomach. Yet, his experiments did not extend to poppy or to opiates.[28] In 1745, however, i.e. three years after the publication of Alston's dissertation, Abraham Kaau Boerhaave (1715–58), physician in The Hague and nephew of Hermann Boerhaave, reported about his own animal experiments, in which he had applied Wepfer's old method in studying the *ratio operandi* of opium. Vivisecting dogs which had been put to deep sleep by high oral doses, he noted that their stomachs still contained the drug after several hours and that the pylorus seemed 'perfectly closed'. In one trial he weighed the remaining amount of opium in the stomach six hours after application and found that the original dose of thirty grains had been reduced by less than one grain. Accordingly Boerhaave supported the view that opiates acted by primarily affecting the nerves of the stomach (and from hence the whole nervous system), i.e. not via absorption and the blood circulation.[29]

So, in principle there were two arguments forming the basis of the theory of an immediate nervous action of opium: first, the clinical observation of a very short interval between ingestion and first effects, which made it seem unlikely that a considerable part of the drug had already been absorbed; and secondly, the experimental observation that opium caused its characteristic narcotic effect, before it was dissolved to a larger extent and before a major part of it had reached the guts, i.e. the place of absorption.[30] A third argument, again based on animal experimentation, was provided in the 1750s by Alston's Edinburgh colleague Robert Whytt (1714–66), Professor in the Institutions of Medicine.[31]

Whytt compared the effects of opium on intact frogs with those on such frogs in which he had previously either excised the heart or cut off the head and destroyed the spinal cord. Thus he experimented on three 'animal models' (as one would say today): one, in which the blood circulation had been stopped, another, in which the central nervous system had been eliminated, and a third, in which both systems worked. Whytt observed that opium – injected into the stomach and the guts – destroyed sensibility and motion in a frog whose heart had been excised as soon as in an intact one. Moreover, he noted that opium applied to muscles or into the body cavities of frogs without a central nervous system diminished the heart-beats much more slowly than it did in entire animals.[32] These findings seemed to show that the nervous system was much more important for bringing forth the effects of opium than the circulatory system. Therefore Whytt endorsed Alston's theory of the drug's direct effect on the extremities of nerves at the site of administration. With regard to intravenous injection of opiates he suggested that the symptoms were due to action on nerves terminating at the internal surface of the heart and the vascular system or on the cerebral medulla itself.[33]

Thus in the middle of the eighteenth century the 'nerve theory' (as it might briefly be called) began to supersede the theory of rarefaction of the blood. Turgid blood vessels in animals poisoned with opium – once an important argument in favour of the latter theory – were now explained as resulting from the reduced and finally stagnating circulation, as demonstrated under the microscope by Alston.[34] Furthermore, Whytt's experiments supporting the 'nerve theory' doubtlessly showed the highest degree of sophistication that had hitherto been reached in this field of research. He had not only compared the effects of opium on specially prepared frogs with intact ones. In true control experiments he had also studied the physiological changes produced by the very process of preparation (i.e. extirpation of the heart, decapitation, and pithing) without application of the drug.[35] Nevertheless it was Whytt's experimental design that soon provoked criticism by still another Edinburgh professor, the anatomist Alexander Monro secundus (1733–1817).

In a paper read before the Edinburgh Philosophical Society in 1761 Monro spoke of an 'unlucky deception' in the chief of the experiments performed by his medical colleague: since the heart-beat continued in decapitated and pithed frogs, Whytt was led to believe (Monro explained) that the opium was still absorbed and mixed with the circulating blood in these animals. Monro, however, had observed microscopically that the blood flow stagnated in the small vessels of such frogs, and he had demonstrated experimentally that absorption became inconsiderable as the circulation ceased. So, in consequence of his wrong presupposition, Whytt had attributed the slow effect of opium in decapitated and pithed frogs only to the lack of a central nervous system, forgetting to take diminished absorption into account here as well. Thus he had generally overestimated the role of the nerves and underestimated the role of absorption in producing the effects of the drug.[36]

Monro therefore used modified animal models, so to speak. Like Whytt he experimented on three different groups of frogs: in a first group he either excised the heart or separated the hind legs preserving only the sciatic nerves as a connection with the trunk. By applying subcutaneously a water solution of opium to the hind legs he hoped to record the pure nervous action of the drug, since the blood circulation had obviously been interrupted in these models. In a second group he either destroyed the lower spinal cord or separated the hind legs preserving only a connection consisting of blood vessels and concomitant lymphatics. Again applying opium to the legs Monro used such animals as models for the study of effects which were brought about solely via absorption and transport in the blood and lymph. And in a third group he applied the solution of opium to the hind legs of intact frogs. Comparing the intensity of systemic drug effects, and the time until their onset, between these three groups, he noted that general symptoms of intoxication were much more intense in the models of pure absorption than in the nerve models, and that they appeared most quickly in the intact animals. Based on these results Monro enlarged the current theory on the mode of action of opium. In his view the effects

were produced both directly through the nerves and by way of absorption into the blood stream.[37] He was all the more convinced of this
modified theory, since he had found in further animal experiments that
alcohol and camphor seemed to act even chiefly via absorption.[38] Yet,
his enlarged theory was still dominated by the idea of opium's immediate action on nerves: like Whytt he maintained that – once absorbed
into the circulating blood – the drug would affect nerves terminating at
the inner side of the heart and of vessels.[39] The second step of rejecting
the 'nerve theory' altogether in favour of the theory of absorption was
taken only twenty years later by the renowned Abbé Felice Fontana
(1730–1805).

In frogs Fontana had carefully laid bare the sciatic nerves of both
sides. On one side he had then dipped the nerve in an aqueous solution
of opium and on the other side in pure water. Since the capacity of these
nerves to conduct stimuli to the muscles of the hind legs decreased in the
same way and to the same extent on both sides, he concluded that
opium had generally no direct effect on nerves. Since, on the other
hand, intravenous injection of opium (in rabbits) caused the known
effects, it followed – in his opinion – that the drug could act only by way
of the blood circulation.[40] Though Fontana had used not less than 300
frogs in the above-mentioned experiments, the evidence produced by
them was rather weak, as was already observed in his own time. A
Göttingen medical student, who had repeated and varied these experiments, confessed in 1789 that he had to smile, when he thought more
deeply about the matter. The natural places for sensation of stimuli
were specially adapted nervous surfaces, he explained. Therefore it was
methodically wrong to apply opium to nervous cords covered by 'thick
cellular' coats, as the 'famous *Fontana*' and he himself had done.[41]
Alexander Monro had made the same point with respect to correspond-
ing experiments of his own already in 1761.[42]

Though contemporary experimental evidence in favour of opium's
direct effect on nerves was certainly stronger than that in favour of the
theory of absorption and transport of the drug in the blood circulation,
it was the latter view that was eventually confirmed in the following
century. As has been suggested by Melvin P. Earles, theories of the
mode of action of drugs and poisons underwent a *general* change from
the later eighteenth to the middle of the nineteenth century, in which
the 'nerve theory' was superseded by the theory of absorption. Essential
for this change, according to Earles, were physiological studies in the
early nineteenth century, which demonstrated that absorption was not
only performed by the lymphatics but also immediately – and thus
quickly – by veins, and which provided insight into the high speed of

the circulation. Moreover, nineteenth-century toxicologists succeeded in identifying poisons in the blood and in the tissues of organs, a fact which also helped to discredit the 'nerve theory' and to strengthen the view that drug effects were brought about by way of absorption.[43] The eighteenth-century research on opium that I have described seems to foreshadow this forthcoming general change in pharmacological theory, or, more precisely, it seems to have contributed to this change in a very early stage.

Effects on cardiac activity

Besides the *modus operandi* of opium, its effects on heart activity were a subject of particular scientific interest in the second half of the eighteenth century. In his famous paper on 'sensible and irritable parts', read to the Göttingen Royal Society of Sciences in 1752, Albrecht von Haller (1708–77) had stated that opium destroyed the peristaltic movements of the guts and almost all irritability (i.e. contractility) throughout the body, while the motions and force of the heart were not impaired by it in the least.[44] Haller founded this assertion on some vivisections of opiated frogs and dogs, which he had carried out in the preceding year together with his pupil Johann Adrian Theodor Sproegel (1728–1807).[45] Their findings, however, contrasted sharply with those of Whytt. Having administered opium in various ways to the same kinds of animals the Edinburgh professor recorded a significant deceleration of the heart-beats, sometimes ending with total cardiac arrest.[46] In particular he observed that the heart rate decreased sooner in frogs which had been given opium than in frogs which had been decapitated and pithed. Furthermore, the contractions of excised frogs' hearts stopped sooner if they had been immersed in a water solution of opium than if immersed in pure water.[47]

As usual in the eighteenth century, a scientific dispute developed. Somewhat maliciously Whytt wrote in 1755 that Haller's 'candor and love of truth' would certainly 'make him readily acknowledge his mistake, as soon as he shall discover it'.[48] Haller retorted by arguing that Whytt's very invasive vivisectional procedures created artificial conditions, which rendered his observations worthless:[49] 'Ouvrir le ventre d'un animal, lui couper la tête ou la moelle de l'épine, pour connoitre les effets plus ou moins lents d'un poison, n'étoit surement pas le moyen d'apprendre la vérité.'[50] Haller did not seem to realize, however, that the same objection could as well be made against his and Sproegel's experiments. Moreover, he apparently ignored that Whytt had made control experiments.

Monro sided with Whytt, yet Haller quoted experiments of Fontana supporting his position.[51] What at first glance looks like a quarrel about a minor problem concerning the pharmacology of opium was actually a central issue of the so-called Haller–Whytt controversy over sensibility and irritability.[52] The two opponents agreed that opium diminished and finally destroyed sensibility. If this effect was associated with a decrease of the heart rate, and thus a diminution of the irritability of the heart, Whytt's doctrine that irritability depended on sensibility would have been strengthened. If, on the other hand, the motions of the heart continued without any change, this would have given support to Haller's theory that irritability (or contractility) was an independent, specific property of muscle fibres, enduring in the absence of any nervous influence.[53]

The debate stimulated other researchers to make trials on human beings, including themselves. Yet the results were as divergent as they had been in the initial animal experiments. In 1764 Maxwell Garthshore (1732–1812) stated in his Edinburgh inaugural dissertation, which was partly based on experiments on himself, that opium taken in a moderate dose accelerated the blood circulation, while it otherwise diminished irritability, relaxed the muscles, and caused sleepiness. Already in the next year, however, the young Samuel Bard (1742–1821), student of the same university, reported in his doctoral thesis that his own pulse count as well as that of three friends and six convalescents had decreased significantly after taking the moderate dose of one and a half grains.[54] Haller himself took up the issue again in 1776 by giving an account of his personal experiences with opium enemas, which he used regularly over a long period in the treatment of his own final illness. He had found that his pulse count increased after the pain-relieving clysters, and he regarded this as confirmation of his earlier view that irritability was independent from sensibility.[55]

In retrospect, one will first tend to assume that these differing observations were – apart from the problem of artefacts – simply due to different doses of opium. Yet, this problem was seen quite clearly, at least by Haller, who repeatedly emphasized that very high doses, which ultimately killed an animal or man, of course diminished and finally destroyed cardiac activity.[56] A problem, however, which was not recognized clearly enough in this debate, and which could not be solved in the eighteenth century, was the varying contents of active substances in the drug. It was not certain whether the customary crude opium, chiefly imported from Turkey, Egypt, and East India, was really the pure dried juice of slit poppy capsules, or whether it contained the weaker meconium, i.e. the pressed and dried juice of the whole plant, or

whether even other drugs might have been admixed.[57] In the absence
of exact methods of standardization and before the isolation of morphine (F. W. Sertürner 1804) and other effective substances,[58] differing
observations of the pharmacological effects of opium, and thus controversies, were probably inevitable.

Still, towards the end of the eighteenth century some answers to the
riddle asked by Haller and Whytt were tried. The German physician
Carl Joseph Wirtensohn (d. 1788) suggested in his doctoral thesis in
1775, that 'opium weakens the fibres of the heart, yet increases the
movement of the blood', because it diminished the irritability or contractility of the blood vessels and thus the resistance of the vascular
system.[59] The aforementioned Göttingen medical student who had
criticized Fontana – Georg Christoph Siebold (1767–98), son of the
Würzburg Professor of Anatomy, Surgery and Obstetrics Carl Caspar
Siebold – further elucidated the role of dosage. In a prize essay on the
effects of opium on the healthy body, published in 1789, he derived a
general rule from several experiments on warm- and cold-blooded
animals: in moderate doses an initial increase of the heart rate is
followed by a decrease, and the higher the dose the shorter the period of
this transitory acceleration of the pulse.[60] Samuel Crumpe (1766–96),
an Irish physician, came independently, yet four years later, to a similar
result by counting his own and a healthy test person's pulse after taking
usual therapeutic doses of one to two and a half grains of opium. The
pulse rate – measured in five minutes intervals over one or two hours –
first went up, but then dropped to its initial level or somewhat below.[61]
Both Siebold and Crumpe integrated these experimental findings into a
general 'two stages'-concept of the clinical effects of opium. The rise of
the pulse belonged to the first stage characterized by alacrity and
hilarity, increased transpiration and respiration, whereas its fall was
part of the second stage characterized by painlessness, lethargy, sleepiness, and impeded respiration.[62]

Crumpe, who also cited the results of his own animal experiments as
confirming this concept, interpreted the two stages of the drug's effect
in terms of the Brownian system: opium as a stimulant raised the degree
of excitement and in this way caused sthenia in the first stage. The
second stage was the consequence of exhausted excitability and thus
represented a state of so-called indirect asthenia.[63]

Brownian physicians hailed Crumpe's work as experimental proof of
their therapeutic system. The German Brownian Melchior Adam
Weikard (1742–1803) published an enthusiastic review of Crumpe's
study in his *Magazin der verbesserten theoretischen und praktischen Arzneikunst*:
'After the experiments made in this work there cannot be any doubt

any longer that opium is a stimulant. The relief of pain follows only a previous stimulus, an increase of pain etc. Thus opium diminishes sensibility, if it has induced indirect asthenia . . . Almost everything goes together with Brown's doctrine.'[64] Conversely, from the party of those physicians who held to the view that opium was a sedative, Crumpe's experiments and conclusions were rejected. The latter had found, for example, both in animal and in self-experimentation, that a water solution of opium applied to the eye caused pain and inflammation, and he had taken this as an indication of the drug's stimulating effect.[65] A critic, however, pointed out, that this observation was worthless, because 'every extraneous body' would cause pain, if applied to the eye, and in many instances even pure water would produce this effect.[66]

The example of Crumpe's work sheds some light on contemporary points of contact between experimental research on opium and its therapeutic use in medical practice. Thus it brings up the question of which concrete contributions to current problems in opium therapy were made by experimentalists, and what medical practitioners thought about these contributions.

Applied research

A matter of dispute in eighteenth-century pharmacotherapy was the efficiency of external, topical application of opium. As mentioned above, Alston had not seen any effect in his experiments on himself. In the next decades the problem was repeatedly taken up by other experimentalists. Monro compared the effects of a water solution of opium after internal administration and external application to frogs. He observed the same effects in both cases, yet their onset was quicker, if the drug had been given internally, and he therefore recommended that opium should be taken orally, even if pain or convulsions were localized.[67] John Leigh (before 1755–after 1792), an American physician who did some experimental work on opium at the University of Edinburgh in the 1780s, repeated Alston's trials with opium plasters on two men. Since he too saw no effects, he concluded that 'the common received opinion respecting the operation of opium, externally applied, must be erroneously founded'.[68] Crumpe confirmed Alston's and Leigh's findings on his own skin.[69] Siebold, however, observed several effects in dogs, which he had rubbed with an ointment of opium, including pollakiuria, sleepiness, and typical changes of the pulse, and he reported that he had even killed a naked, new-born rabbit by immersing its body into a strong solution of the drug.[70] Thus there was a discrepancy between the results of animal experiments, which suggested that externally applied opium had some effect, and experiments on human beings, which seemed to prove that this form of administration was ineffective.

Though the results of applying opium experimentally to human skin were unambiguously negative, medical practitioners did not seem to think of giving up external therapy. For instance, a reader of Leigh's study wrote unimpressed in the *Critical Review* in 1786: 'Dr. Leigh found the external application of opium had little effect; yet, whoever has tried it in spasmodic pains of the side, in hysteric affections of the stomach, or . . . in a locked-jaw, will probably find it a useful remedy.'[71] Case reports about the successful treatment of delirious states with embrocations of opium were quoted as an argument in favour of external therapy.[72] And as late as in 1803 a German Brownian physician affirmed in Ernst Horn's *Archiv für medizinische Erfahrung* that embrocations of opium had proved useful in 'asthenic pains of all kinds of diseases'.[73]

In a related field of opium therapy experimentally gained results were equally ignored. It was customary in the eighteenth century to combine caustics with opium in order to alleviate the pain caused by the former. Alston had already doubted that this procedure was useful, yet had not made a test.[74] Monro, however, demonstrated that solutions of opium applied to the skin of frogs were unable to prevent the intensive pain caused by a later application of the caustic spirit of hartshorn (*Spiritus cornu cervi*).[75] Nevertheless, the admixture of opium to caustic mercurial preparations, usually employed in the treatment of venereal diseases, was still recommended in the early nineteenth century.[76]

Further examples for the quite disapproving attitude towards results of applied research on opium can be observed with regard to some other findings of John Leigh. Based on chemical and pharmacological experiments – the latter made partly on animals, partly on some test persons of different ages and sex, and a few patients – Leigh had shown that the resin of opium was the most efficient part, that a mixture of the resin with extract of liquorice was most quickly dissolved in the stomach, and that previous ingestion of acids lessened the effects of the drug.[77] Yet, the critic of the *Monthly Review* claimed that Leigh had not made any new observations,[78] and his colleague on the *Critical Review* maintained that the experiments were 'few, trifling, and inconclusive'.[79] The latter particularly faulted the varying effects on different test persons and demanded 'an extensive series of trials'. But even this would only be a first step, because the diseases changed the effects of the drug. Therefore this critic rather recommended the observations of the 'more attentive practitioners'.[80] This response leads to the question what the above-mentioned two eighteenth-century authorities on opium therapy, the practitioners Young and Tralles, thought about contemporary experimental research on opium.

It is remarkable that both of them expressed their disapproval towards experimental endeavours. Young rejected chemical experiments with drugs, since remedies revealed their medical effects in the human body – not in the retort. He did not accept *in vitro* trials on freshly let blood, because this blood was not any longer continually changed by absorption and secretion. Moreover, he did not acknowledge the results of intravenous injections in animals, for even harmless milk had acted as a deadly poison, when applied in this way. And an examination of a drug by recording its smell and taste could, in his opinion, merely give some first clues about its properties. Young therefore trusted only in practical experiences with opium in the treatment of various diseases.[81] Similarly Tralles declared that he was not ready to give up his belief in opium's stimulating effect on the blood circulation, simply because Whytt had come to different conclusions through some experiments on frogs. The Breslau physician assured that he had convinced himself of this effect in thousands of patients in many years of medical practice. Nobody could expect from him that he should set greater store by 'marshy frogs' than by his therapeutic experience.[82]

Evidently the problem of transferability of pharmacological findings in lower animals to diseased human beings played a role here. It was generally discussed in this time, also with respect to experimentation in physiology.[83] Particularly Monro was well aware of this kind of difficulty, asserting that the *intensity* of the effects of opium was of course different in frogs and men, but not the basic *mode* of action.[84] Yet, the question of transferability was certainly not the only problem in this context. As the described reactions to experimental research on opium suggest, a general distrust in the new pharmacological approach to remedies seems to have existed among eighteenth-century physicians: if experimental findings disagreed with therapeutic practice, they were ignored or rejected; if they agreed, they were dismissed as being nothing new.

Still, towards the end of the eighteenth century a more friendly attitude towards pharmacological research on opium can be traced as well. A critic of Leigh's study wrote in the *Medicinische Bibliothek*, a review journal edited by the Göttingen Professor of Medicine Johann Friedrich Blumenbach (1752–1840):

The trials which the author has made with opium . . . are always interesting, yet in the whole, and particularly in comparison with the almost innumerable, divergent and often contradictory trials of his many predecessors, still not sufficient to draw reliable general conclusions. If only someone had the wit, knowledge and time to perform a truly pragmatic revision of all these hitherto published trials, to repeat the most decisive of them, to compare them etc., so that this now still mainly dead capital might have some practical use at last.[85]

It is quite possible that it was Blumenbach himself who had written these lines, for in the same year, 1788, he initiated and formally put a prize question on the effects of opium to the students of the Göttingen medical faculty.[86] The study of Siebold discussed above was the only work that came in, and it won the prize, yet not for this reason alone. The medical faculty praised Siebold for his high number of careful animal experiments and his prudent and cautious conclusions drawn from them.[87] Blumenbach published a very positive review of the prizewinning essay in the *Göttinger Gelehrte Anzeigen*. He particularly emphasized the student's findings concerning the relation between dose of opium and pulse rate and stated that the 'useful practical conclusions and applications' included in this work gave an example of the 'important, immediate beneficial use' that practical medicine gained from theoretical inquiries of this kind.[88] In fact Siebold had advised, for example – on the basis of his experimental results – to give small doses of opium, if the pulse and other vital functions of a patient had to be increased, and to administer larger doses, if patients needed sedation.[89] Thus at least in the case of Siebold's work on opium a first step towards the recognition of experimental pharmacology as the basis of pharmacotherapy seems to have been made.

PSYCHOPHARMACOLOGICAL OBSERVATIONS

Though seventeenth- and eighteenth-century scientific interest in opium was chiefly directed towards its bodily effects, psychic changes after the taking of the drug were not left unrecorded. The Paris pharmacist and physician Moyse Charas (1619–98), for example, who did a few self-experiments in the late seventeenth century, repeatedly noted a strongly tranquillizing effect, occasionally accompanied by insomnia. He did not elaborate on this, however, since he was predominantly interested in the gastrointestinal effects of opium.[90] Much more attention was paid to the psychological effects by John Jones, who actually eulogized them: opium

causes a brisk, gay and good Humour . . . Promptitude, Serenity, Alacrity, and Expediteness in Dispatching and Managing Business . . . Assurance, Ovation of the Spirits, Courage, Contempt of Danger, and Magnanimity . . .

prevents and takes away Grief, Fear, Anxieties, Peevishness, Fretfulness . . . causes Euphory, or easie undergoing of all Labour, Journeys, &c. . . . lulls, sooths, and (as it were) charms the Mind with Satisfaction, Acquiescence, Contentation, Equanimity, &c.[91]

Jones listed all these effects in an effort to discredit the traditional seventeenth-century theory that opium acted by diminishing or disabling the animal spirits, and in order to substantiate his own theory of opium causing primarily a 'pleasant Sensation' (see above). The basis of his knowledge were mainly reports on habitual opium taking from travellers to Oriental countries, though he also stated that 'some who tried it among us, have found it so'. Jones probably wrote from his own experience as well, and he compared the effects of opium – as did many later authors – with those of 'generous Wine'.[92]

Still, in the course of the eighteenth century it was argued that those euphoric effects might be seen in the inhabitants of the Orient, who were accustomed to the use of the drug, but could not be expected in unaccustomed persons in the western world.[93] Against the background of this criticism self-experiments by western doctors gained importance. John Leigh included a report of such an experiment, sent to him by his friend Dr James Ramsay from Virginia, when he published his own experimental work on opium in 1786.[94] Six years later the same report was quoted again *in extenso* by Samuel Crumpe.[95] Ramsay described in detail what he experienced one night after taking Thebaic Tincture (i.e. a solution of opium in alcohol and cinnamon water). He first noticed an enlivening effect, which enabled him to continue studying. A second, greater dose – to counteract 'a violent drowsiness coming on' – led to a state of exhilaration that made him careless of his works and expressed itself in 'excesses of dancing, singing, &c.'. Ramsay now noted a strong pulse, impaired sight, vertigo, and difficulties in walking. Gone to bed he lay 'almost motionless', feeling unable to move: 'my imagination was so distressed by the appearance of horrid images, that I could not close my eyes till seven, when I fell into an interrupted slumber'.[96] Crumpe basically confirmed Ramsay's observations in his own experiments on himself. He experienced from large doses of opium 'an increased flow of spirits, an observable gaiety, cheerfulness, and alertness, which, subsiding into a state of pleasing languor, terminated ultimately in a degree of drowsiness, stupor, and disinclination to motion'. Crumpe's test persons showed and reported 'the same effects'.[97]

Neither Ramsay nor Leigh provided a pharmacological theory to explain the psychic changes. Crumpe remained within his general Brownian framework by attributing the first, euphoric stage to stimulation and the second, stuporous stage to exhausted excitability or indirect asthenia.[98] Yet these early self-experiments introduced a basic method of psychopharmacology: taking a defined dose of a drug, careful self-observation, and detailed recording of mental and physical symptoms. In the nineteenth century this method began to be used in a more systematic way, e.g. by the Grenoble physician and scientist Pierre-Alexandre Charvet (1799–1879), whose Paris dissertation of 1826, *De l'action comparée de l'opium, et de ses principes constituans sur l'économie animale*, has recently been labelled as 'the first book on modern experimental psychopharmacology'.[99] At about the same time self-observation after taking of drugs was presented in a fashionable manner to a larger readership through Thomas de Quincey's *Confessions of an English Opium-Eater* (1st edn, 1821).[100]

In comparison with contemporary experimentation aiming at the purely physical effects of opium, and particularly when compared to the carefully designed experiments that were made in studying the intake of the substance into the body, the few eighteenth-century psychopharmacological trials may appear rather crude. This must not only be attributed, however, to a secondary interest in the psychic effects of the drug. Whereas physiology provided a methodical basis for the former, somatic type of experimentation, no specific tools were available in the eighteenth century to carry out a thorough psychological examination of drug effects.

ETHICAL ASPECTS

As is evident from the sources discussed in this chapter, eighteenth-century pharmacological studies on opium were mainly based on animal experimentation and to a lesser extent on experiments on human beings. Since it was known that the debate on vivisection had its origins in the seventeenth and eighteenth centuries, it seemed promising to look for ethical considerations in those sources.[101] For two obvious reasons, however, only a few relevant remarks can be found in the examined works on opium: first, as a narcotic opium mitigated – at least in high doses – the usual suffering of vivisected animals. In fact one occasionally finds a short comment that an opiated experimental animal showed no or only few signs of pain during vivisection.[102] Secondly, since opium was a frequently prescribed remedy, the transition from its therapeutic use to its scientific test on human beings was quite smooth.

With respect to animal experimentation Haller's pupil Sproegel included some utterances of compassion in his protocols. For instance, he remarked that – after poisoning with opium and vivisection – he finally strangled 'the poor dog'; or he noted with regard to another poisoned dog: 'At last we released it from its tortures.' Yet, this releasing was nothing else but death through vivisection.[103] A similar tinge of compassion can also be traced in Siebold. In the preface to his prize essay he assured that it was only 'just' that he had also experimented on himself, for he had 'tortured' so many animals.[104] Crumpe excused the 'apparent inhumanity' of his animal experiments by their necessity in studying 'many points among the most interesting to mankind'. He furthermore stated that he was not ready to sacrifice animals in trials with highly concentrated extracts of opium, because this would be an unnecessary cruelty, particularly since such experiments would have no therapeutic consequences.[105] Such remarks were characteristic of contemporary attitudes of experimentalists to the suffering of their animals. They reflected some degree of sensibility, but no serious moral concern. In view of a possible increase of medical knowledge and improvements of therapy animal suffering was held to be easily excusable. Compassion was generally no major obstacle to experimental work on living animals.[106]

With regard to human experimentation some concern not to endanger the test person's health is expressed within the studies of both Crumpe and Leigh.[107] Yet the standards as to which effects of the drug were reasonable for the experimentees to bear seem to have been quite low. Leigh reported, for instance, that he 'got two patients in the same room', on whom he tried the comparatively high dose of five grains of resin and gum of opium. In the patient who had received the resin – a thirty-year-old man – the symptoms 'increased to so violent a degree as to cause a kind of raving', and the other who had been given the gum – a twenty-five-year-old woman – was 'affected with violent convulsions'. Leigh did not write a word about possible therapeutic purposes connected with these trials. Just to the contrary, he explained that these experiments had been made 'with a view to discover, whether there was any difference in the operation of the resinous and gummy parts of opium'.[108] In the protocol of another trial Leigh confessed that only with some difficulty he prevailed on a healthy man to take some drops of a presumedly very effective solution of oil of opium. It brought on such vehement vomiting that it deterred Leigh from making any further experiments of this kind.[109] Impressive as such reports may appear to the modern reader, in order to put them into a proper perspective, however, one has to keep in mind that researchers who experimented with opium on human beings, such as Leigh and Crumpe, did not exclude themselves from the group of test persons.[110]

Particularly the latter experiment of Leigh suggests that at least in some cases the risks of a trial were discussed with the test person beforehand. Yet, it would certainly not be appropriate to speak of informed consent in a modern sense[111] in these eighteenth-century trials.

CONCLUSIONS

The first experimental studies in the pharmacology of opium – carried out in the eighteenth century – followed three main lines. First, they tried to elucidate the basic mode of action of the drug. *In vitro* and animal experiments here brought about changes of relevant theories. The iatromechanical doctrine that opium rarefied the blood was superseded by the theory of the drug's direct effect on nerves, which in turn was questioned by the view that it was absorbed and conveyed with the blood to its sites of action. The latter transition seems to reflect an early stage of a general change in pharmacological theory. The second line of research, dealing with the effects of opium on heart activity, played a crucial role in the study of sensibility and irritability, and thus in an important area of eighteenth-century physiology. Experiments on animals and human beings eventually led to a 'two stages'-concept of the clinical effects of opium, which helped to overcome earlier controversies. Experimentation devoted to concrete questions of opium therapy, representing the third line of research, was generally not acknowledged by medical practitioners. They clearly set greater store by their own therapeutic experiences with opiates than by the results of the new pharmacological approach. Besides those main lines, a few self-experiments made by doctors in the late eighteenth century were devoted to the psychic changes caused by opium. Careful self-observation and recording of symptoms were introduced as a basic method of psychopharmacology. Finally, as for the ethics of animal and human experimentation with opium, it has been observed that neither compassion with experimental animals nor a certain concern not to harm the test persons prevented extensive and sometimes dangerous trials.

ACKNOWLEDGEMENTS

Research for this chapter was begun at the Institut für Geschichte der Medizin of the University of Göttingen and completed during a Wellcome Fellowship at the Wellcome Institute for the History of Medicine in London. I would like to thank the Trustees of the Wellcome Trust for their support and for providing excellent research facilities. Moreover

I owe special thanks to Marlies Glase and the late Dr Frank W. P. Dougherty, Göttingen, for their kind assistance in examining archive material on Siebold's prize essay, and to Professor Roy Porter, London, for his helpful comments on an earlier draft of this chapter.

NOTES

1 J. C. Kramer, 'Opium Rampant: Medical Use, Misuse and Abuse in Britain and the West in the 17th and 18th Centuries', *British Journal of Addiction*, 74 (1979), pp. 377–89; M. Kreutel, *Die Opiumsucht* (Stuttgart, 1988), pp. 154–204.

2 See as a representative work: George Young, *A Treatise on Opium, Founded upon Practical Observations* (London, 1753). See also A. N. Bindler, 'Schmerz und Schmerzbehandlung zwischen 1650 und 1760. Eine Untersuchung anhand von Dissertationen aus dem deutschen Sprachraum' (Med. Diss., Basel, c. 1986), p. 26; M. Seefelder, *Opium. Eine Kulturgeschichte*, 2nd edn (Munich, 1990), pp. 125f.

3 See Kramer, 'Opium Rampant', pp. 380f; M. M. Weber, 'Die "Opiumkur" in der Psychiatrie. Ein Beitrag zur Geschichte der Psychopharmakotherapie', *Sudhoffs Archiv*, 71 (1987), pp. 31–61.

4 J. Brown, *The Elements of Medicine . . . Translated from the Latin, with Comments and Illustrations, by the Author. New Edition, Revised and Corrected. With a Biographical Preface by Thomas Beddoes*, 2 vols. (London, 1795), I, pp. xxiii, 107f, II, pp. 14f.

5 A. Ch. H. Henke, 'Abhandlung über die Wirkungsart und klinische Anwendung des Mohnsafts, mit Hinsicht auf die Meinungen der älteren, neueren und neuesten Zeit über diesen Gegenstand', *Archiv für medizinische Erfahrung*, 4 (1803), pp. 765–839; G. B. Risse, 'The Brownian System of Medicine: Its Theoretical and Practical Implications', *Clio Medica*, 5 (1970), pp. 45–51; *idem*, 'Brunonian Therapeutics: New Wine in Old Bottles?', in W. F. Bynum and R. Porter (eds.), *Brunonianism in Britain and Europe* (*Medical History*, Supplement No. 8, London, 1988), pp. 46–62; V. Jantz, 'Pharmacologia Browniana. Pharmakotherapeutische Praxis des Brownianismus aufgezeigt und interpretiert an den Modellen von A. F. Marcus in Bamberg u. J. Frank in Wien' (Pharm. Diss., Marburg an der Lahn, 1974), pp. 208–36; Th. Henkelmann, *Zur Geschichte des pathophysiologischen Denkens. John Brown (1735–1788) und sein System der Medizin* (Berlin, Heidelberg, and New York, 1981), pp. 5, 49; H. J. Schwanitz, *Homöopathie und Brownianismus 1795–1844. Zwei wissenschaftstheoretische Fallstudien aus der praktischen Medizin* (Stuttgart and New York, 1983), pp. 62–5.

6 G. Sonnedecker, 'Emergence of the Concept of Opiate Addiction', *Journal Mondiale de Pharmacie*, 5 (1962), pp. 275–90, and 4 (1963), pp. 27–34; Kramer, 'Opium Rampant', pp. 385–7; Kreutel, *Opiumsucht*, pp. 158–80.

7 J. Jones, *The Mysteries of Opium Reveal'd*, 2nd edn (London, 1701), pp. 36–9. A typical supporter of this old theory was the Jena Professor of Medicine Georg Wolfgang Wedel (1645–1721); see his *Opiologia ad mentem Academiae Naturae Curiosorum* (Jena, 1674), pp. 40f.

8 Jones, *Mysteries*, pp. 92–8, 207–34.

9 *Ibid.*, pp. 315–18.

10 Jakob Descazals, *De opiatorum nova eaque mechanica operandi ratione . . . sub Praesidio*

. . . *Dn. Friderici Hoffmanni* (Halle, 1700), pp. 20f; Christoph Fimmler, *De vi opii rarefaciente, a qua, ostenditur, omnia illius effecta in homine proficisci, Praesidio D. Io. Gothofredi Bergeri* (Wittenberg, 1703), pp. 12f; see also Richard Mead, 'A Mechanical Account of Poisons', in *The Medical Works*, 3 vols. (Edinburgh, 1765), I, pp. 1–158, on pp. 132f. He combined the two theories of pleasant sensation and rarefaction of the blood.

11 Young, *Treatise on Opium*, pp. 25–7, 32, 140–3; B. L. Tralles, *Usus opii salubris et noxius, in morborum medela, solidis et certis principiis superstructus*, 4 parts (Breslau, 1757–62), pt 1, pp. 80–4, 171–6, pt 2, pp. 80f, 123f.

12 Henke, 'Abhandlung über die Wirkungsart', p. 772.

13 See Paul Scheel, *Die Transfusion und Einsprützung der Arzeneyen in die Adern* (Copenhagen, 1802), pp. 36f, 40, 45, 50, 206–8, 211f; H. Buess, *Die historischen Grundlagen der intravenösen Injektion* (Aarau, 1946), p. 145 and *passim*.

14 R. Boyle, 'Of the Usefulness of Natural Philosophy', in *The Works*, 5 vols. (London, 1744), I, pp. 423–554, on p. 479.

15 J. S. Elsholtz, *Clysmatica nova*, 2nd edn (Berlin, 1667; repr. Hildesheim, 1966), pp. 14–16; Scheel, *Transfusion*, pp. 206–8, 211f.

16 H. Sloane, 'Experiments and Observations of the Effects of Several Sorts of Poisons upon Animals, etc. Made at Montpellier in the Years 1678 and 1679, by the Late William Courten Esq.', *Philosophical Transactions*, 27 (1712), pp. 485–500. Toxicological tests with opium, administered orally to two dogs and a cat, were also reported by the Danish botanist and chemist Ole Borch (1626–90); see Scheel, *Transfusion*, p. 187.

17 J. W. Estes, 'John Jones's Mysteries of Opium Reveal'd (1701): Key to Historical Opiates', *Journal of the History of Medicine and Allied Sciences*, 34 (1978), pp. 200–9.

18 Sloane, 'Experiments', pp. 493f.

19 Mead, 'Mechanical Account', p. 133; J. Freind, *Emmenologia* (Rotterdam and Leiden, 1711), p. 168; Fimmler, *De vi opii*, p. 15.

20 Mead, 'Mechanical Account', pp. 136f; Fimmler, *De vi opii*, pp. 9–11; Freind, *Emmenologia*, pp. 176, 178, 184f. For Freind's *in vitro* experiments see also M. Lindenberger, 'Pharmakologische Versuche mit dem menschlichen Blut im 18. Jahrhundert' (Dent. Med. Diss., Berlin, 1937), pp. 9–14.

21 Freind, *Emmenologia*, pp. 172f; Mead, 'Mechanical Account', pp. 135f; Fimmler, *De vi opii*, pp. 12–14.

22 Ch. Alston, 'A Dissertation on Opium', *Medical Essays and Observations*, 5 (1742), pt 1, pp. 110–76.

23 *Ibid.*, pp. 153–5, 160f, 171. Paradoxically, Alston writes that his *in vitro* trials 'agree perfectly with Dr. *Freind*'s Experiments (*Emmen.*, c. 14)'.

24 *Ibid.*, p. 159. On the supposed external efficiency of opium see e.g. Jones, *Mysteries*, pp. 17f, 207f.

25 M. P. Earles, 'Experiments with Drugs and Poisons in the Seventeenth and Eighteenth Centuries', *Annals of Science*, 19 (1963), pp. 241–54; K. Schöpf, 'Der Schlaf aus medizinischer Sicht im 18. und frühen 19. Jahrhundert' (Med. Diss., Munich, 1987), pp. 72–5.

26 Alston, 'Dissertation on Opium', pp. 165–70.

27 See A.-H. Maehle, *Johann Jakob Wepfer (1620–1695) als Toxikologe* (Aarau, Frankfurt a.M. and Salzburg, 1987), pp. 117–20. Wepfer was quoted by Alston, 'Dissertation on Opium', pp. 165f.

28 See Maehle, *J. J. Wepfer*, pp. 72–6, 80–6, 91–3.

29 A. K. Boerhaave, *Impetum faciens dictum Hippocrati per corpus consentiens philologice et physiologice illustratum observationibus et experimentis passim firmatum* (Leiden, 1745), pp. 401–7.

30 It must be considered in this context that according to contemporary doctrine absorption was performed chiefly – if not completely – by the lymphatic system, i.e. that the drug had to be absorbed by the chyle vessels of the guts and transported the long way through the thoracic duct, before it entered the blood of the subclavian vein. See N. Mani, 'Darmresorption und Blutbildung im Lichte der experimentellen Physiologie des 17. Jahrhunderts', *Gesnerus*, 18 (1961), pp. 85–146; *idem*, *Die historischen Grundlagen der Leberforschung* (Basel and Stuttgart, 1967), pp. 84–103; M. P. Earles, 'Early Theories of the Mode of Action of Drugs and Poisons', *Annals of Science*, 17 (1961), pp. 97–110.

31 See also R. K. French, *Robert Whytt, the Soul, and Medicine* (London, 1969), pp. 50–3.

32 R. Whytt, 'An Account of Some Experiments Made with Opium on Living and Dying Animals', *Essays and Observations, Physical and Literary*, 2 (1756), pp. 280–316.

33 *Ibid.*, pp. 302–4. See also R. Whytt, 'An Essay on the Vital and Other Involuntary Motions of Animals', in *The Works*, publ. by his Son (Edinburgh, 1768), pp. i–viii, 1–208, on pp. 199f.

34 *Idem*, 'Account', p. 313.

35 *Ibid.*, pp. 281–5.

36 A. Monro, 'An Attempt to determine by Experiments, how far some of the most powerful Medicines, viz. Opium, ardent Spirits, and essential Oils, affect Animals by acting on those Nerves to which they are primarily applied, and thereby bringing the rest of the Nervous System into Sufferance, by what is called Sympathy of Nerves; and how far these Medicines affect Animals, after being taken in by their absorbent Veins, and mixed and conveyed with their Blood in the Course of its Circulation; with Physiological and practical Remarks', *Essays and Observations, Physical and Literary*, 3 (1771), pp. 292–365, on pp. 299–302.

37 *Ibid.*, pp. 336–9, 360–2.

38 *Ibid.*, pp. 340–58.

39 *Ibid.*, pp. 364f. See also A. Monro, *Experiments on the Nervous System with Opium and Metalline Substances* (Edinburgh, 1793), p. 16.

40 Felice Fontana, *Traité sur le Vénin de la Vipère, sur les Poisons Américains, sur le Laurier-Cerise et sur quelques autres Poisons Végetaux*, 2 vols. (Florence, 1781), II, pp. 358–64. See also P. K. Knoefel, *Felice Fontana Life and Works* (Trento, 1984), pp. 290–2.

41 Georg Christoph Siebold, *Commentatio de effectibus opii in corpus animale sanum maxime respectu habito ad eius analogiam cum vino* (Göttingen, 1789), p. 82.

42 Monro, 'Attempt', pp. 325f.

43 See M. P. Earles, 'Studies in the Development of Experimental Pharmacology in the Eighteenth and Early Nineteenth Centuries' (PhD thesis, University of London, 1961), pp. 368–418; *idem*, 'Early Theories', pp. 103–10.

44 A. von Haller, *Von den empfindlichen und reizbaren Teilen des menschlichen Körpers*, ed. K. Sudhoff (Leipzig, 1932), p. 46.

45 See J. A. Th. Sproegel, *Dissertatio inauguralis medica sistens experimenta circa varia venena in vivis animalibus instituta* (Göttingen, 1753), pp. 25–42, 70–4; A. von Haller, *Mémoires sur la Nature Sensible et Irritable, des Parties du Corps Animal*, 4 vols. (Lausanne, 1756–60), I, pp. 331–5, 339, 371f, 386.

46 Whytt, 'Essay', pp. 197f; *idem*, 'Observations on the Sensibility and Irritability of the Parts of Men and other Animals', in *Physiological Essays* (Edinburgh, 1755), pp. 97–223, on pp. 200–13; *idem*, 'Account', pp. 305f.

47 *Ibid.*, pp. 282–91, 293–7.

48 Whytt, 'Observations', p. 213.

49 A. von Haller, 'Reponse à la Critique de M. Whytt', in *idem*, *Mémoires*, IV, pp. 99–133, on pp. 126, 129f.

50 *Ibid.*, p. 131. See also A. von Haller, *Elementa physiologiae corporis humani*, 8 vols. (Lausanne and Berne, 1757–66), V, p. 609.

51 See Monro, 'Attempt', pp. 320f, 332; Haller, 'Reponse', pp. 130f; Fontana, *Traité*, II, p. 342.

52 See also French, *R. Whytt*, pp. 52f, 73.

53 Whytt, 'Essay', p. 198; Haller, 'Reponse', pp. 127f.

54 See Maxwell Garthshore, *Dissertatio medica inauguralis, de papaveris usu, tam noxio, quam salutari in parturientibus, ac puerperis* (Edinburgh, 1764); Samuel Bard, *Tentamen medicum inaugurale, de viribus opii* (Edinburgh, 1765). Both were quoted by B. L. Tralles, *Ad Illustri Viri Christian Gottlieb Ludwigii . . . Disquisitionem de vi opii cardiaca adversariis medico-practicis insertam humanissima responsio* (Breslau, 1771), pp. 23f. For a summarizing review of Garthshore's thesis see *Göttinger Anzeigen von gelehrten Sachen*, no. 152 (1765), p. 1224, and of Bard's see *Mediciinschchirurgische Bibliothek*, 4 (1777), pp. 247–50.

55 A. von Haller, *Abhandlung über die Wirkung des Opiums auf den menschlichen Körper*, ed. E. Hintzsche and J. H. Wolf (Berne, 1962), pp. 5–8, 11, 16f.

56 *Ibid.*, pp. 5f; Haller, 'Reponse', pp. 128f.

57 Alston, 'Dissertation on Opium', pp. 111–24; [Paul Scheel], 'Zusätze und Anmerkungen des Uebersetzers', in Samuel Crumpe, *Auf Versuche gegründete Untersuchung der Natur und Eigenschaften des Opiums* (Copenhagen, 1796), pp. 193–216, on pp. 194f.

58 See J. C. Kramer, 'The Opiates: Two Centuries of Scientific Study', *Journal of Psychedelic Drugs*, 12 (1980), pp. 89–103.

59 C. J. Wirtensohn, *Dissertatio medica inauguralis demonstrans opium vires fibrarum cordis debilitare et motum tamen sanguinis augere* (2nd edn, Münster, 1775), pp. 20–4.

60 Siebold, *Commentatio*, p. 22.

61 S. Crumpe, *An Inquiry into the Nature and Properties of Opium; Wherein its Component Principles, Mode of Operation, and Use or Abuse in Particular Diseases, are Experimentally Investigated; and the Opinions of Former Authors on These Points Impartially Examined* (London, 1793), pp. 33–5. See also Jantz, 'Pharmacologia Browniana', pp. 215–23.

62 Siebold, *Commentatio*, pp. 7–11, 20–3; Crumpe, *Inquiry*, pp. 192f.

63 Crumpe, *Inquiry*, pp. 98f, 184f, 192f.

64 *Magazin der verbesserten theoretischen und praktischen Arzneikunst*, I (1796), p. 166. The translation is mine.

65 Crumpe, *Inquiry*, pp. 24f, 54, 169.

66 *Critical Review; or Annals of Literature*, 11 (1794), p. 68.

67 Monro, 'Attempt', pp. 303–9.

68 J. Leigh, *An Experimental Inquiry into the Properties of Opium, and Its Effect on Living Subjects* (Edinburgh, 1786), pp. 96–8.

69 Crumpe, *Inquiry*, pp. 27f.

70 Siebold, *Commentatio*, pp. 37f.

71 *Critical Review; or Annals of Literature*, 62 (1786), p. 132.

72 See 'Ward über den äusserlichen Gebrauch des Mohnsaftes' and 'Ebendesselben, neuere Bemerkungen über den äusserlichen Gebrauch des Mohnsaftes', in *Sammlung auserlesener Abhandlungen zum Gebrauche praktischer Aerzte*, 19 (1800), pp. 275–98.

73 Henke, 'Abhandlung über die Wirkungsart', p. 825.

74 Alston, 'Dissertation on Opium', pp. 159f.

75 Monro, 'Attempt', pp. 327f.

76 Henke, 'Abhandlung über die Wirkungsart', p. 836.

77 Leigh, *Experimental Inquiry*, pp. 29–72, 86–125.

78 *Monthly Review; or, Literary Journal*, 76 (1787), p. 258. In fact animal experiments with different solutions and extracts of opium – in order to study the relative efficacy of its components – had already been carried out in the late seventeenth century. See Ole Borch, *De somno et somniferis maxime papavereis dissertatio* (Copenhagen and Frankfurt, 1682), pp. 25–8; Samuel Schroeer, *Disputatio inauguralis de opii natura et usu* (Erfurt, 1693), pp. 8, 11. Experiments on dogs with the resinous and gummy parts of opium had been made in the first half of the eighteenth century by Caspar Neumann (1683–1737) in Berlin and by Christian Wilhelm Schwartz, a student of Andreas Büchner (1701–69), in Magdeburg. See Schwartz, *Dissertatio inauguralis medica de genuinis opii effectibus in corpore humano* (Magdeburg, 1748), and Earles, 'Studies', p. 160.

79 *Critical Review; or Annals of Literature*, 62 (1786), p. 132.

80 *Ibid.*

81 Young, *Treatise on Opium*, pp. 4–13.

82 Tralles, *Ad . . . Ch. G. Ludwigii . . . Disquisitionem*, p. 25.

83 A.-H. Maehle, *Kritik und Verteidigung des Tierversuchs: Die Anfänge der Diskussion im 17. und 18. Jahrhundert* (Stuttgart, 1992), pp. 15–44.

84 Monro, 'Attempt', pp. 294f.

85 *Medicinische Bibliothek*, 3 (1788), p. 56. The translation is mine.

86 See Universitätsarchiv Göttingen, Medizinische Fakultät, Dekanats- und Promotionsvorgänge 1788. See also the forthcoming edition of Blumenbach's correspondence by F. W. P. Dougherty.

87 Universitätsarchiv Göttingen, Med. Fak., Dek.- u. Prom. 1789; Ch. G. Heyne, *Opuscula academica collecta et animadversionibus locupletata*, 6 vols. (Göttingen, 1785–1812), IV, pp. 110f.

88 *Göttingische Anzeigen von gelehrten Sachen*, no. 29 (1790), pp. 281–3.

89 Siebold, *Commentatio*, p. 11.

90 See C. Salomon-Bayet, 'Opiologia, imposture et célébration de l'opium', *Revue d'Histoire des Sciences*, 25 (1972), pp. 125–50.

91 Jones, *Mysteries*, pp. 21f.

92 *Ibid.*

93 Cf. Crumpe, *Inquiry*, p. 45.

94 Leigh, *Experimental Inquiry*, pp. 113–17.

95 Crumpe, *Inquiry*, pp. 46–8.
96 Ramsay as quoted in Leigh, *Experimental Inquiry*, pp. 113–16.
97 Crumpe, *Inquiry*, pp. 45f.
98 *Ibid.*, pp. 192f.
99 R. K. Siegel and A. E. Hirschman, 'Charvet and the First Psychopharmacological Studies on Opium: A Historical Note and Translation', *Journal of Psychoactive Drugs*, 15 (1983), pp. 323–9. A short thesis on the basis of the dissertation was submitted by Charvet to the Paris Faculty of Medicine for the degree of medical doctor; see P.-A. Charvet, *Propositions sur l'action de l'opium chez l'homme et les animaux* (Paris, 1826). Summarizing the main results, this thesis does not discuss the psychological effects of opium, however.
100 See Th. de Quincey, *Confessions of an English Opium-Eater*, 2nd edn (Edinburgh and London, 1856), pp. 195–213.
101 See Maehle, *Kritik und Verteidigung des Tierversuchs*; idem and U. Tröhler, 'Animal Experimentation from Antiquity to the End of the Eighteenth Century: Attitudes and Arguments' in N. A. Rupke, ed., *Vivisection in Historical Perspective*, 2nd edn (London and New York, 1990), pp. 14–47.
102 See e.g. Sproegel, *Dissertatio*, pp. 26, 29, 35, 37; Whytt, 'Account', p. 299.
103 Sproegel, *Dissertatio*, pp. 31, 35.
104 Siebold, *Commentatio*, p. 4.
105 Crumpe, *Inquiry*, pp. 54, 77.
106 See Maehle, *Kritik und Verteidigung des Tierversuchs*, pp. 86–96.
107 Crumpe, *Inquiry*, p. 77; Leigh, *Experimental Inquiry*, p. 57.
108 Leigh, *Experimental Inquiry*, pp. 110–12.
109 *Ibid.*, pp. 56f.
110 See *ibid.*, pp. 87f, 100f; Crumpe, *Inquiry*, pp. 24–8, 33–6, 65–8, 80–2.
111 See R. R. Faden, T. L. Beauchamp and N. M. P. King, *A History and Theory of Informed Consent* (New York and Oxford, 1986).

FOUR

THE REGULATION OF THE SUPPLY OF DRUGS IN BRITAIN BEFORE 1868

S. W. F. HOLLOWAY

THE regulation of the supply of drugs became the subject of a lively debate in Britain during the second half of the nineteenth century. The basic question underlying this debate was, who should determine the availability of drugs in society, consumers, producers, or officials? From these discussions, three distinct models of regulation can be constructed: consumer sovereignty, occupational control, and bureaucratic regulation. By adding a local/national dimension to these categories, a six-fold classification can be produced. Within consumer sovereignty, a distinction can be made between the nationwide, individualistic, free-market model of the classical economists and the local, popularist, communal model of the democratic radicals. The subtypes of occupational control are based on the difference between regulation by local guilds and that by national professional associations. Similarly, regulation by local and central government can be distinguished. This classification is not intended as an analytic, conceptual typology of drug regulation but merely as a rough-and-ready sorting device. Its aim is the understanding of specific historical events and conditions, not the creation of logical, rational, universal theories.

The practice of pharmacy by the apothecary from the mid-sixteenth to the mid-eighteenth century obtained its characteristic features from origins in the medieval urban economy. The guild system with its strict control over who might practise a given craft, who might be trained, how one was to be trained, and how the craft was to be practised, provided the framework within which the apothecary operated. Craft guilds have been subject to widely different assessments.[1] From Adam Smith onwards, economists have generally regarded them as imposing irrational fetters on individual enterprise and free trade, as self-regarding groups opposed to the interests of the consumer and of society at large. Others, who have doubted the beneficence of market forces, have seen them as agents of social solidarity and economic morality. R. H. Tawney, as befits a socialist economic-historian, combined both interpretations. The guilds were, he wrote, 'first and foremost, monopolists, and the cases in which their vested interests came into collision with the consumer were not a few'. Nonetheless, the guilds claimed, at least, to subordinate economic interests to social needs, in an era in which the social and the spiritual were inextricably intertwined. Tawney believed that some virtue might be found in the guilds' attempts

to preserve a rough equality among 'the good men of the mistery', to check economic egotism by insisting that every brother shall share his good fortune with another and stand by his neighbour in need, to resist the encroachments of a conscienceless money-power, to preserve professional standards of training and craftsmanship, and to repress by a strict corporate discipline the natural appetite of each to snatch special advantages for himself to the injury of all.[2]

In late medieval and early modern Europe, craft guilds were formed specifically to oversee and regulate the activities of all practitioners of a particular craft, or group of crafts, within the region controlled by the town. Guilds combined juridical, political, religious, and recreational functions but the economic function of protection against external competition from other towns and regions, and of regulation of internal competition for raw materials and customers within the craft, was crucial. The guilds constituted a *via media* between total monopoly and unrestricted competition, offering a measure of security while at the same time allowing individual effort to be rewarded. The craft guilds sought to maintain a steady volume of business for their members, to guarantee a high standard of workmanship and to obtain a fair or 'just' price for its products. They also tried to restrict the number of apprentices a master might keep, the hours he might work, and the tools he could use. The line between protection and exploitation for both producers and consumers was often blurred. Yet Sylvia L. Thrupp maintains that 'direct evidence of price policies in a local industry, or of their success, is rare' and that 'evidence that points to restrictive policies . . . is seldom conclusive'.[3] The demise of the guild system was brought about, not by disgruntled consumers, but by frustrated producers. And while it prospered, its supervision of training through the apprenticeship system produced a cadre of skilled craftsmen, whose discipline, self-esteem, and pride in their work, were significant factors in the development of European manufacture and technology.

Abundant evidence reveals the existence of organized commerce in the supply of drugs in the principal urban areas of England from at least the fourteenth century. Leslie Matthews, the doyen of British historians of pharmacy, noted that 'a complete list of those engaged in handling drugs and spices, for during the medieval period the trade was frequently combined, would fill many pages'.[4] In a series of articles, he traced the development of the sixteenth-century apothecary from the spicer of the fourteenth century to the grocer of the fifteenth century in the towns of York, Leicester, Norwich, and Canterbury. In York, the Fraternity of the Blessed Mary became in 1408, the Guild of Corpus Christi, which, in turn, was incorporated in 1581, into the wealthy Merchant Adventurers' Company, which comprised mercers, grocers, ironmongers, and apothecaries. In Leicester apothecaries were in a large guild of merchants, while in Norwich they were, in 1561, associated with physicians and barber-surgeons, but after civic reorganization in 1622, they were relegated to the fourth company which comprised upholders, tanners, and other trades. In Canterbury the apothecaries joined a fellowship of grocers, chandlers, and fishmongers. In Salisbury, a Merchants' Company, renamed the Grocers' Company in 1613, consisted of apothecaries, grocers, mercers, goldsmiths, linen-drapers, milliners, vintners, upholsterers, and embroiderers. In Chester there was a composite guild of mercers, ironmongers, grocers, and apothecaries and in Lichfield the all-embracing guild was simply known as the Mercers' Guild. Only London was large and prosperous enough to support separate guilds for most crafts and trades. The setting up of the Society of Apothecaries in 1617 marked the formal separation of the London apothecaries from the Grocers' Company. But, in the city, the Royal College of Physicians tried, from its foundation in 1518, to supervise the activities of the apothecaries. An Act of 1540 gave the College the right to enter the shop of any apothecary, examine his wares, and, if found to be defective, to have them destroyed.[5]

Considerable caution must be exercised before attempting to characterize the early regulation of the retail supply of drugs in England as a form of occupational control. In London, the College of Physicians and the Society of Apothecaries, both occupational associations with government authorization, fought one another for control of the practice not only of pharmacy but also of medicine. Losing ground in the vending and compounding of drugs to the emergent druggist, apothecaries sought new ways of controlling the market for their services by usurping the physician's right to diagnose and prescribe. This shift in the definition of their occupational role was accompanied by a widening of their geographical horizon. In place of the local jurisdiction of the urban guild, they sought to establish a nationwide system of professional regulation. A central authority to guarantee competence and quality of service and to secure a monopoly for qualified practitioners became the main thrust of the movement for medical reform after 1794.

In the provinces, the historical evidence suggests that pharmaceutical practice was supervised by multi-craft guilds. However, so close was the relationship between these guilds and borough government, that it would not be inappropriate to describe such regulation as local authority control. Prosecutions for illegally retailing drugs were instigated by guilds but tried before the mayor and council. Moreover, by no means all urban areas had guilds. By 1689 only a quarter of the 200 towns in England had any form of guild organization.

In his seminal study, *The Political Theory of Possessive Individualism*, C. B. Macpherson has uncovered the novel and fundamental assumptions about man and society which came to permeate political thinking during the seventeenth century and which survive as the infrastructure of liberal theory today. The central feature of this new discourse was the 'possessive quality' of the individualistic approach embedded in seventeenth-century thinking.

Its possessive quality is found in its conception of the individual as essentially the proprietor of his own person or capacities, owing nothing to society for them. The individual was seen neither as a moral whole, nor as part of a larger social whole, but as an owner of himself. The relationship of ownership, having become for more and more men the critically important relation determining their actual freedom and their actual prospect of realising their full potentialities, was read back into the nature of the individual. The individual, it was thought, is free inasmuch as he is proprietor of his own person and capacities. The human essence is freedom from dependence on the wills of others, and freedom is a function of possession. Society becomes a lot of free equal individuals related to each other as proprietors of their own capacities and of what they have acquired by their exercise. Society consists of relations of exchange between proprietors . . . Political society is a human contrivance for the protection of the individual's property in his person and goods, and for the maintenance of orderly relations of exchange between individuals regarded as proprietors.[6]

The theory of possessive individualism legitimized and celebrated the transition from a guild-based to a free-market economy. The guild system had recognized the human value of labour: for Hobbes, it was merely 'a commodity exchangeable for benefit'. Vocation as a fixed status with its own honour was replaced by occupational mobility and the system of exchange. By the eighteenth century, the Physiocrats could proclaim the privileges of guilds as 'contrary to the order of nature'. In 1776, Adam Smith in *The Wealth of Nations* built his conception of the natural economic order on the assumption of possessive individualism.

Adam Smith argued that the guild system led to inefficient deployment of both labour and stock. 'The exclusive privileges of corporations . . . keep up the market price of particular commodities above the natural price, and maintain both the wages of labour and the profits of stock employed about them somewhat above their natural rate'. Guild regulation fails to ensure good workmanship, he asserted, and 'has no tendency to form young people for industry'. 'The real and effectual discipline which is exercised over a workman is not that of his corporation, but that of his customers'. Smith even trotted out the time-worn accusation that 'people of the same trade seldom meet together, even for merriment and diversion, but the conversation ends in a conspiracy against the public, or in some contrivance to raise prices'.[7]

The chemist and druggist was one of the beneficiaries of the collapse of the guild system. The fundamental tenets of his philosophy began with the belief in the unrestricted right of every man to follow whatever occupation was most congenial to his temperament or best calculated to put money in his pocket. Ordinances and statutes which created reserved occupations were repressive because they interfered with the prerogatives of the individual. The regulation of a trade must be left to the sovereignty of the consumer. The need to attract custom, rather than adherence to communal standards, was the driving force behind the activities of the chemist and druggist. He inaugurated a two-fold freedom: his own liberty to dispense whatever pharmaceutical preparation he may wish, to whomever he may wish, without any restriction; and the liberty of the public to purchase and use whatever drug it may choose.[8]

The third quarter of the eighteenth century saw the birth of a consumer society in Britain.[9] Before that century it had not been thought possible that consumers at all levels of society might acquire new wants and find new means of generating purchasing power. 'Consumption is the sole end and purpose of all production', wrote Adam Smith, 'and the interest of the producer ought to be attended to only as far as it may be necessary for promoting that of the consumer. The maxim is . . . perfectly self-evident.' Many truths were found to be self-evident in the eighteenth century which previously had been inconceivable and have since seemed less than obvious.

The emergence of the chemist and druggist was part of the commercialization of British society. He was one of the group of small traders who succeeded in exciting new wants and making available new goods to the eighteenth-century public. By boosting demand, they helped to create a new consumer market of unprecedented size and buying power. Chemists and druggists were busy, inventive, profit-making businessmen, whose eager advertising, active marketing, and inspired salesmanship did much to usher in a new type of society in eighteenth-century England. By 1780 the value of sales of proprietary medicines was estimated at £187,500 a year. In 1783 the government, confident this trade would continue to grow, imposed a stamp tax on it.

The number of chemists and druggists increased markedly in the years after 1780. From that date, not only was there an increase in the absolute number in all the urban areas of Britain but also a growth relative to the rising population and relative to the growing number of other medical practitioners. Chemists and druggists rapidly became established as a new species of *homo medicus*.

The success of the chemist and druggist depended upon his ability to meet his customers' needs. These needs, in turn, were grounded in the old tradition of family self-medication. In pre-industrial Britain the sick person habitually played an active role in interpreting and managing his state of health.[10] Self-diagnosis and therapy were standard practice at all levels of society and the ordinary person regularly dispensed medicine to friends, family, and servants. Laymen believed, with good reason, that they could understand illness and treat it just as effectively as the medical practitioner. In the seventeenth century well-established families prepared their own medicines and kept them ready in the kitchen. By the late eighteenth century middle-class families were starting to stock up with drugs and medicines bought from the chemist and druggist. Both rich and poor made use of his services for the compounding of family recipes. The popularity of manuals of domestic medicine and of family medicine chests indicates the widespread extent of new forms of self-diagnosis and self-medication during the eighteenth century.

The more consumer power fuelled the rise of the chemist and druggist, the more the general medical practitioner sought ways of containing it. The movement for the professionalization of medicine, with its emphasis on the value of specialized training and knowledge, established an assault not only on the freedom of the chemist and druggist but also upon the tradition of family self-medication. The medical reformers, by placing the patient firmly under the doctor's control, would cut out competition from the druggist. The essence of quackery was patient self-help, the practice of medicine beyond the control of the qualified. The free market was seen as a conspiracy between buyer and seller which produced profit-hungry drug sellers and obsequious doctors ingratiating themselves with their clients by giving them what they demanded.[11]

Medical botany was the most significant social movement of the 1840s to express its opposition to the professionalization of medicine by defending the traditional right of everyman to be his own physician. Medical botany was popularized in Britain chiefly by Albert Isaiah Coffin, who arrived in England from New York State in 1838. Coffin was the purveyor of a system of herbal remedies, devised by Samuel Thomson in North America, where it attained considerable popularity in the open, democratic, self-improving culture of the Jacksonian era. Medical botanists believed that all disease could be traced to obstructions in the flow of bodily heat. The obstruction was brought to the surface by the use of *lobelia inflata* (Indian tobacco) which could be used as an emetic or inhaled in hot vapour baths. Medicines made from cayenne pepper (capsicum) restored the flow of heat. 'There is now actually in existence', claimed Coffin, 'a complete system of medical treatment which each individual can take into his own hands with little trouble, and almost without expense – a system at once embracing all that is safe and good in all others known'.

Coffin went on lecture tours in the North of England with the aim of setting up local societies, members of which had to possess his book, *The Botanic Guide to Health*. Coffin tried to secure the active involvement of ordinary people in the organization. The local societies were democratically run with elected committees whose responsibility it was to see that one or more members visited and prescribed for all the sick who sought the help of the society. Another member kept stock of the society's collection of roots and herbs. At each weekly meeting, members reported on their successes and discussed any difficult cases, in order 'that the people may mutually assist each other in the study of Medical Botany'.

Coffinism was a form of popular resistance to the cultural aggression involved in the professionalization of medicine. The professional attitudes and social pretensions of doctors were vigorously attacked:

the licensed to kill enters the house of sickness, and, at the bedside, takes in charge, with the authority of law, his exclusive right over the prostrate victim, whose blood he draws, whose frame he tortures, whose bowels he secretly poisons, and whose disease he cures, or, at his will, prolongs: but kill or cure, his charge is made, in amount wholly at his own discretion.

'Thousands perish under their hands who would otherwise have survived', claimed Coffin. 'Mercury, opium, alcohol, and the use of the lancet are of themselves sufficient to account for the speedy depopulation of a world.'

For centuries the medical profession had been accumulating power but now was the time to 'throw off the yoke of medical despotism'. The people must be released from 'medical bondage'. To achieve this, medical knowledge must be demystified and medical practice deprofessionalized. When stripped of 'the false airs of pedantic learning' there is nothing in medicine beyond the reach of the ordinary mind. It was not 'a difficult, abstruse, mysterious science': it only seemed so because 'the learned have combined together for the purpose of throwing dust into the eyes of the people'. But the system of medical botany had been freed 'from all technicalities' and was 'so easy to be understood that every member of society may learn it if disposed'. Medical botany was the people's medicine: 'the common sense of the people, when in possession of a true theory of medicine, will be found quite capable of curing all diseases to which they are subject'. With the aid of Coffin's *Botanic Guide*, 'every father can now discharge the duties of physician to his own household'.

The essence of medical botany was democratic self-care, i.e. the idea that all human beings are obliged to care for each other. The founding of local societies was to help 'the poorest of his fellow countrymen to help themselves'. Thomsonian practitioners carefully explained the proposed course of treatment to the patient and his friends before proceeding. They believed that medicine was a subject which all should be equally taught and in which the advantages and duties are mutual. Professionalism in medicine is anti-democratic: it involves the privatization of public knowledge. Like the enclosing of the common land, it deprives the ordinary man of his birth-right. 'To mystify, shut up in the schools, and make private property of that knowledge, which of all others ought to be universally taught, is a wrong the deepest and most injurious to society'.

Medical botany had a considerable following among factory operatives, craftsmen, artisans, tradesmen, and small shopkeepers in the North and Midlands. The organization and ideology appealed to intelligent working men, deeply interested in radical politics, religious dissent, and self-improvement. Among them, there was a strong current which rejected the elitism of those in authority and distrusted the services of professionals. This is clearly seen in the continued support for community private venture (common-day) schools long after the provision of publicly subsidised elementary education; in the numbers of adults who attended unpretentious mutual improvement societies rather than the civically approved Mechanics' Institutes; and in the working-class preference for local preachers and an unpaid ministry rather than the 'hireling priests' of the Established Church.

The medical profession was uncompromising in its hostility to Coffinism. Both class and professional interests drove it to track down and prosecute practitioners of medical botany whenever the opportunity arose. The Thomsonian system was recognized as a comprehensive challenge to the established position and the swelling pretensions of the orthodox practitioner. The idea that former cotton-spinners, bricklayers, or stonemasons could become competent to practise medicine with little more instruction than that to be garnered from a few lectures, Coffin's manual and mutual discussion ran directly counter to the orthodox practitioner's demands for prolonging training and tightening qualifying requirements.[12]

The idea of an egalitarian, locally-based, communal control of the supply and use of drugs, such as that envisaged by the followers of Thomson and Coffin, is usually dismissed today as unrealistic. A plausible model for the exercise of community control of pharmacy, it is argued, presupposes a very elementary pharmacopoeia and a simple division of labour in which all work is sufficiently unskilled to be easily learned and performed by everyone. There is no provision in such a model for the complex knowledge systems and the elaborate occupational specialization characteristic of advanced industrial societies. The same objections are used to denigrate attempts to revive the ideals of the medieval guilds. Schemes of participatory democracy in industry, such as those advocated by guild socialists like G. D. H. Cole, are widely regarded as exercises in romantic nostalgia. The guild system was founded upon a system of economic relations which were personal, intimate, and direct. It assumed a level of organization small enough for the moral standards applicable to face-to-face relations to be upheld.

Yet a growing body of opinion and research suggests that there is no single appropriate size for organizations and institutions. Different structures are appropriate for different purposes. The task of matching organizational structures to human values has no predetermined outcome. Modern science and technology do not lead inevitably to large-scale, impersonal, centralized, bureaucratic organizations. Nor is the present social division of labour sacrosanct and unchangeable. Since it was socially constructed, it can be politically deconstructed.

A major feature of the ideology of professionalism has been the emphasis on the individual professional's service to individual clients in a relationship of individual trust. The professional man, it is said, cannot spread his services, cannot go in for mass production, and cannot, except within narrow limits, distribute his skills through subordinates. Traditionally, the essence of professionalism has been found in the belief that the individual is the true unit of service because service depends on individual qualities and individual judgement, supported by an individual responsibility which cannot be shifted on to the shoulders of others.[13] If there is any justification at all for such views, it follows that large-scale corporate agencies, whether run by the state or privately, are just as inimical to professional control as they are to community control. Yet few people today question the right, even the necessity, for professional involvement in the regulation of the supply of drugs. There can surely be little doubt that contemporary methods of regulating the supply of drugs, both nationally and internationally, represent one of the most striking failures of modern public administration. When methods of regulation cause greater social problems than the object of the regulation, a disastrous escalation can only be averted by a fundamental change of direction. In this context, the politics of ecology, with its emphasis on a sustainable economy, decentralization, and the human scale of organizational structures, may seem more visionary than backward-looking.[14]

When the Pharmaceutical Society of Great Britain was founded in 1841, any person in this country could sell and advertise practically any medicine he liked, could put into it whatever he pleased, could call it by any name he fancied and claim for it anything and everything he wished the public to believe. The public were likewise free to buy any drug or pharmaceutical preparation they wished, in any quantity, without restriction from the chemist or the necessity of a medical prescription. Even the physician's prescription implied the minimum of medical control since it belonged to the patient and could be dispensed indefinitely. Since the majority of raw materials were so cheap and the competition among vendors so keen, the most potent substances were obtainable by all bar the destitute. Pennyworths of poison, observed John Simon in 1854, were handed across the counter as nonchalantly as cakes of soap.

The fundamental objective of the Pharmaceutical Society was to become the regulatory authority for pharmacy in Britain. The intention was to take the amorphous, inchoate mass of individual chemists and druggists and mould it, by the leadership of the metropolitan elite, into a self-respecting profession which commanded the confidence of the public. The leading pharmaceutists saw themselves not as mere

shopkeepers retailing goods at competitive prices but as skilled practitioners selling their services. The public relied upon their knowledge
and skill in manufacture, compounding, and dispensing. Their specialist knowledge of drugs was required to provide the basis for determining
their purity and freshness, for recommending them for their efficacy in
treating illness, for furnishing advice on their dosage and mode of
administration, and for warning of their dangers. Since the customer
placed his health and even his life in the chemist's hands, specialist
knowledge and experience, honesty, reliability, and integrity were of
vital importance.

The task of the Pharmaceutical Society was to substitute the corporate reputation of a professional organization for the individual repu-
tations of practitioners as the basis of public trust. The Society would
achieve this by rooting out the charlatans and the incompetent, by
exercising surveillance over the activities of its members, by drawing up
a code of ethics, and by controlling the entry, education, examination,
and registration of future practitioners.

The organisation of a body of chemists into a society, the chief objects of which
are avowedly to raise the character of the profession of pharmacy, and to
ensure a uniform and efficient administration of medicine, will confer upon
every member, that public confidence to which he is entitled. It will be in the
power of the society to inculcate the impolicy of adulterations, to enlighten the
public mind as to the mischief of cheap medicines, and thus to overcome to a
great extent the prejudice which exists amongst too many of us in favour of a
mistaken economy, and also to disseminate the advantages of that scientific
knowledge which every druggist ought to possess.[15]

More than a year before the foundation of the Pharmaceutical
Society, the editors of *The Chemist* had argued that: 'The retail chemist
ought . . . to be compelled to undergo a strict examination as to his
knowledge of the nature of drugs and their medical properties, so as to
enable him to detect any error in prescription and insure his committing no mistake through ignorance.'[16]

Jacob Bell, the editor of the *Pharmaceutical Journal*, pointed out that:

The society was established for the purpose of . . . raising the character of those
who practice pharmacy in Great Britain. It is proposed to attain this end, first,
by uniting all the chemists and druggists into one body; secondly, by introducing a system of pharmaceutical education; thirdly, by claiming for the body
thus organised and educated, such protection and privileges as the qualifications of the members would entitle them to possess.[17]

'The chemists, having until lately been disunited, and ranked rather
with the trades than the professions', wrote Bell ten years later, 'have

not had the advantage of that discipline which is the natural result of organisation and professional intercourse.'[18]

The founding of the Pharmaceutical Society was not the outcome of a growing sense of professional solidarity and consciousness among chemists and druggists. Its establishment was an attempt by a small elite of London dispensing chemists 'to take the government of their body into their own hands'. Their plan was to regulate and control the rest of the profession. When the Society tried to persuade its members to place professional responsibility and public service above self-interest, when it inveighed against price competition and short-sighted profiteering, when it condemned chemists and druggists for their ignorance and incompetence and disowned them for practising as apothecaries, it was promoting the interests of the metropolitan elite against the immediate interests of other sections of the trade. It is not surprising that many chemists and druggists declined to join. They had no pretensions to become professional men. They were not eager to acquire commercially irrelevant qualifications, nor to pay an annual levy to a remote London corporation. Above all, they did not welcome the prospect of having their work subjected to inspection and surveillance. Those who have to submit to discipline find its merits less obvious than those who administer it. The majority of chemists and druggists wanted to be left alone to carry on making money. 'Not only does Free Trade secure the public the best at the lowest cost', they argued, 'but by the same law of operation it provides and encourages the best talent, the highest skill, and the greatest experience'.[19]

As a voluntary association, the Pharmaceutical Society found itself with an inescapable double-facing stance. Janus-headed, it promised its members protection and progress, but, at the same time, spoke of regulation and control. It first needed sufficient members to establish itself as a financially viable, permanent, and representative association. It wanted to make good its claim to speak for the pharmaceutical body as a whole. Unless it offered protection and advancement it risked having no members at all. On the other hand, it had to make itself acceptable to powerful groups in the medical profession and to the representatives of public opinion. To its putative sponsors, therefore, it spoke of discipline, regulation, and control.

The only effective resolution of this dilemma was the intervention of the state. The professionalization of pharmacy required the sanction of the legislature, the supreme legitimizing and enforcing institution. 'At the time that the Pharmaceutical Society was founded', claimed Jacob Bell in 1844, 'an Act of Parliament was the ulterior object to which the chemists aspired.'[20]

We have always maintained that our body is and must be considered a branch of the medical profession, and that whatever regulations, respecting education, registration or protection, may be considered necessary for medical practitioners, the same or similar enactments are no less requisite in our department . . . It would be absurd to lay great stress on the importance of science and skill in writing the prescription, and at the same time to leave the preparation of it to chance . . . the safety of the public is as much concerned in the suppression of unqualified dispensers of medicine as it is in the suppression of unqualified medical practitioners.[21]

When Jacob Bell introduced his Pharmacy Bill in the House of Commons in 1851 he made clear the need for compulsory powers:

According to the present arrangements, the examination of candidates by the Society was a voluntary matter; and, accordingly, if a person presented himself for examination, and he was found to be incompetent and unfit to receive a certificate, he might commence business without one, ignorant though he were, and could snap his fingers at the examiners . . . It was the object of the Pharmaceutical Society, in introducing the Bill, to make the examination obligatory.[22]

The Society was entirely of a voluntary character; its powers did not extend beyond its own members . . . consequently the influence of the Society numerically on those entering the business was small . . . It was, therefore, necessary, in order to extend that beneficial influence, to increase the powers of the Society, and for this purpose the Pharmacy Bill was introduced.[23]

When the 1851 Pharmacy Bill was considered by a Select Committee, evidence of the regulation of pharmacy overseas was adduced in its support. On the Continent, it was claimed, chemists are all highly educated men. Governments provide schools of pharmacy where students 'have the opportunity of obtaining all the information which the present age of discovery can afford; and they are compelled to undergo a strict examination before they can establish themselves in business'.[24] 'In France the laws', Jacob Bell pointed out,

are so stringent that no person is permitted to give medical advice in the most trivial cases, without possessing a qualification and a licence. A chemist is prohibited from preparing any recipe or prescription for a patient, unless written by a medical man; and no person can carry on the business of a chemist and druggist without having undergone an examination, neither can he employ an assistant who is not qualified.

In Norway, Sweden, Denmark, Finland, Russia, and Germany

not only are unqualified persons prohibited from practising in any department of the profession but the number of regular practitioners is limited by law; only so many being licensed as are considered to be required by the populations in their respective districts . . . The course of education is definite and complete; and the examinations, through which each candidate must pass, are very severe . . . the profession enjoys a monopoly which is rigidly maintained.[25]

The Pharmaceutical Society regarded the dispensing of physicians' prescriptions as the core of the pharmaceutical role. The curriculum of its School of Pharmacy and the syllabus of its examinations were based on this definition of the proper sphere of activity of the pharmaceutical chemist. All other activities, including the sale of poisons, were considered as, at best, ancillary and, more often, distracting. The primary objective of the Society's parliamentary activity in the nineteenth century was to secure for its members a monopoly of the right to compound the prescriptions of physicians and surgeons. In moving the second reading of his Pharmacy Bill in 1851, Jacob Bell explained that:

the object of the measure was to improve the qualifications of pharmaceutical chemists, and to establish the principle, that all those who were to compound the prescriptions of physicians and surgeons ought to receive a certain amount of education, and pass an examination, as a test of their fitness for the performance of their important and responsible duties.

Similarly, the Pharmaceutical Society's Bill of 1864 provided that: 'It shall not be lawful for any person to carry on the business of a chemist and druggist in the keeping of open shop for the compounding of prescriptions of duly qualified medical practitioners in any part of Great Britain unless such person shall be a pharmaceutical chemist.'[26]

Although the leaders of the Pharmaceutical Society recognized that the moral panic about the unrestricted availability of poisons during the 1850s 'led irresistibly to the consideration of the subject of Pharmacy', they consistently opposed the government's schemes to control the sale of poisons by bureaucratic regulation. Nor did they seek legislation which would brand them as 'authorised sellers of poison'. The Pharmaceutical Society's position was that the most effective safeguard in the supply of poisons to the public was the creation of a profession of dispensing chemists.

As at present there is absolute free trade in poisons, *and in medicines generally*, we consider that the first step to be taken is to commence a register of all persons at present dealing in poisons and to enact a law that in future no unregistered person should be permitted to sell *certain classes of medicine* which might be enumerated in a schedule of poisons; and that, after a certain date, all persons dealing in these substances, and *dispensing prescriptions for the sick*, shall be required to pass an examination . . . That we consider would be the most efficient security to the public against accidents from poisons and against criminal poisoning also.[27]

Moreover, although the leaders of the Pharmaceutical Society were not averse to making comparisons with European arrangements when it suited their purpose, they were not seeking to replicate the centralized bureaucratic control of pharmacy found on the Continent. However much they admired the scientific education, professional status, and commercial protection of the French *pharmacien* and the German *Apotheker*, the British chemist and druggist had no desire to be placed under the control of either the medical profession or the state. The pharmaceutical chemist wanted to be in control of his own affairs.

If Pharmacy is to advance and prosper in this country, it must be under the fostering care and management of the Pharmaceutical body. If any science, art, or profession is to be well governed, it must be entrusted to its own members – those who by education, experience, and daily pursuits, are identified with its progress, and acquainted with its requirements. No other profession is subjected to extraneous jurisdiction and interference, and why should Pharmacy be a solitary exception?[28]

The Pharmaceutical Society wanted a state-enforced monopoly in order to protect itself against interference from the state. In mid-Victorian Britain this was not an outrageous request: one of the main responsibilities of the state was recognized to be that of limiting its own activities.

'No industrial economy', comments Dr H. C. G. Matthew in his authoritative biography of W. E. Gladstone, 'can have existed in which the state played a smaller role than that of the United Kingdom in the 1860s.'[29] The relationship between government and civil society was, it was widely believed, 'a marriage of convenience rather than a marriage of true minds'.[30] The aim of government was not to determine the structure and working of society but to provide a framework of rules and guidelines designed to enable society very largely to run itself. In his Budget speech of 1860, Gladstone put it in this way:

in legislation of this kind, you are not forging mechanical supports and helps for men, nor endeavouring to do for them what they ought to do for themselves; but you are enlarging their means without narrowing their freedom, you are giving value to their labour, you are appealing to their sense of responsibility, you are not impairing their temper of honourable self-dependence.[31]

The British prided themselves on the fact that their constitution had so little in common with the more coercive and *étatist* regimes of continental Europe. They rejoiced that Britain had no significant corps of salaried officials but relied, instead, in both central and local government, on the largely unpaid services of the aristocracy. The state, in

Britain, was regarded as an institution of secondary importance. It existed mainly to serve the convenience and protect the rights of individuals in private life. In contrast, civil society, comprising business, work, religion, leisure, culture, and family life, was seen as the highest sphere of human activity. When mid-Victorian governments did intervene in this arena, their involvement had to be justified in strictly functional and expedient terms.

In John Stuart Mill's classic essay *On Liberty*, he warns of the dangers to the freedom of the individual of increasing government intervention. There is in the world, he writes,

an increasing inclination to stretch unduly the powers of society over the individual, both by the force of opinion and even by that of legislation: and as the tendency of all the changes taking place in the world is to strengthen society, and diminish the power of the individual, this encroachment is not one of the evils which tend spontaneously to disappear, but, on the contrary, to grow more and more formidable . . . unless a strong barrier of moral conviction can be raised against the mischief, we must expect, in the present circumstances of the world, to see it increase.[32]

Mill was unable to raise a strong barrier of moral conviction against state regulation of the sale of poisons. Indeed, he discovered good reasons why, in this instance, the powers of society should be increased. Characteristically, he begins by affirming his faith in Free Trade. It is now recognized, he says,

that both the cheapness and the good quality of commodities are most effectually provided for by leaving the producers and sellers perfectly free, under the sole check of equal freedom to the buyers for supplying themselves elsewhere. This is the so-called doctrine of Free Trade, which rests on grounds different from, though equally solid with, the principle of individual liberty asserted in this Essay.

But, 'trade is a social act. Whoever undertakes to sell any description of goods to the public, does what affects the interest of other persons, and of society in general; and thus his conduct, in principle, comes within the jurisdiction of society'.

The sale of poisons raises a new question, that of 'the proper limits of what may be called the functions of police; how far liberty may legitimately be invaded for the prevention of crime, or of accident'. It is, argues Mill, 'one of the undisputed functions of government to take precautions against crime before it has been committed, as well as to detect and punish it afterwards'. Since totalitarian police-states operate on this very principle, it is not surprising that Mill expresses unease at this point.

The preventive function of government, however, is far more liable to be abused, to the prejudice of liberty, than the punitory function; for there is hardly any part of the legitimate freedom of action of a human being which would not admit of being represented, and fairly too, as increasing the facilities for some form or other of delinquency.

Nevertheless, Mill reasserts that, in principle, a public authority may intervene to prevent crime. Similarly, 'it is a proper office of public authority to guard against accidents'. However, when there is not a certainty but only a danger of accident, the individual should 'be only warned of the danger, not forcibly prevented from exposing himself to it'. Mill then turns to the sale of poisons 'to decide which among the possible modes of regulation are or are not contrary to principle'. 'If poisons were never bought or used for any purpose except the commission of murder, it would be right to prohibit their manufacture and sale. They may, however, be wanted not only for innocent but for useful purposes, and restrictions cannot be imposed in the one case without operating in the other.'

That, one might suggest, goes without saying. Mill then turns to specific proposals.

Such a precaution, for example, as that of labelling the drug with some word expressive of its dangerous character, may be enforced without violation of liberty: the buyer cannot wish not to know that the thing he possesses has poisonous qualities. But to require in all cases the certificate of a medical practitioner, would make it sometimes impossible, always expensive, to obtain the article for legitimate use.

Mill ignores here the view put forward by both doctors and chemists that patients might understandably be reluctant to swallow medicine labelled poisonous. The case for having educated sellers of poisons was to provide the purchaser of drugs with reassurance and guidance about dosage, since toxicity and effectiveness were closely related. But Mill ignores the pharmaceutical aspect of poisons and treats the problem solely as a police matter. For him the issue is to find ways of preventing crime 'without any infringement, worth taking into account, upon the liberty of those who desire the poisonous substance for other purposes'. Mill's preoccupation with liberty leads him to make recommendations that are simply bureaucratic.

The seller, for example, might be required to enter in a register the exact time of the transaction, the name and address of the buyer, the precise quality and quantity sold; to ask the purpose for which it was wanted, and record the answer he received. When there was no medical prescription, the presence of some third person might be required, to bring home the fact to the purchaser, in case there should afterwards to reason to believe that the article had been applied to criminal purposes.[33]

There was nothing original in Mill's discussion of the sale of poisons. His proposed solution was already standard practice. As early as the 1840s, two local Acts of Parliament, for Manchester and Stockport, had prohibited the sale of arsenic and prussic (hydrocyanic) acid to anyone under the age of twenty-one and to anyone else, except in the presence of two witnesses, and provided that various details of the purchases were entered in a poisons book. The Arsenic Act of 1851 was the first attempt by the central government to restrict, on a national scale, the sale of poison. By that Act retailers of arsenic were required (1) to sell only to adults (2) to mix the arsenic with soot or indigo (3) to enter in a book the name, address, and occupation of the purchaser, the date of the sale, the quantity sold, and the purpose for which required (4) unless the purchaser were known, to sell only in the presence of a witness known to both parties and (5) to ensure that the entry was signed by the seller, the purchaser, and, where necessary, the witness.

With no provision for its enforcement, the Arsenic Act was more a declaration of intent than an effective piece of legislation. Yet, by the time John Stuart Mill was completing the drafts of his famous essay, the British government was proposing to extend the provisions of the Act to other poisons. An increasing number of poisons were being used not only in medicine but in arts, manufacture, and agriculture. People in many walks of life required access to them, not only for self-medication, but also in the household, workshop, and field.

During the years 1857–9 the Pharmaceutical Society successfully opposed the governments' attempts to solve the poisons question by detailed regulations. 'The security of the public', argued Jacob Bell, 'would be better effected by an attention to the intelligence and qualification of the vendor than by any arbitrary regulations.' The sale of poisons is an activity which requires the exercise of judgement and discretion. Detailed regulations would take away 'from the pharmaceutical chemist, the person who sells the poison, that responsibility which at present is a great safeguard to the public'.

In a recent article, Dr Peter Bartrip has argued that the 1851 Arsenic Act was 'a first legislative step towards pharmaceutical reform. Indeed, it presaged the Pharmacy Act of 1852 and the much more important Pharmacy and Poisons Act, 1868.' 'With the passage of the Arsenic Act', he continues, 'the close association between poisons and pharmaceutical regulation was established.'[34] This view seems to place undue emphasis on the mere fact of chronology. There was, and is, a world of difference between the mode of regulating the sale of drugs advocated by the Pharmaceutical Society and that enshrined in the Arsenic Act. It is the difference between professional and bureaucratic forms of control. The 1851 Act and the Poisons Bills of 1857–9 were attempts by the state to regulate the sale of poisons *without* becoming involved in the reform of pharmacy. Throughout the nineteenth century, British governments declined to accept responsibility for the promotion of pharmaceutical science, education, and practice. Their sole concern in promoting poisons legislation was the prevention of crime. And in that, perhaps, lies the cause of all our present woes. A fervid concern for the liberty of the individual has produced, on an international scale, a bureaucratic regulation of the supply of drugs in which the rights of individuals, and even of nations, are systematically violated.

NOTES

1 Antony Black, *Guilds and Civil Society in European Political Thought from the Twelfth Century to the Present* (London, 1984), chs. 1–2.

2 R. H. Tawney, *Religion and the Rise of Capitalism* (Harmondsworth, 1938), pp. 39–40.

3 Sylvia L. Thrupp, 'The Gilds', in M. M. Postan, E. E. Rich, and E. Miller, eds., *The Cambridge Economic History of Europe*, vol. III (Cambridge, 1963), ch. 5, pp. 230–80.

4 Leslie G. Matthews, *History of Pharmacy in Britain* (Edinburgh, 1962), pp. 37–40.

5 J. G. L. Burnby, *A Study of the English Apothecary from 1660 to 1760* (London, 1983).

6 C. B. Macpherson, *The Political Theory of Possessive Individualism* (Oxford, 1962), pp. 3, 264.

7 Black, *Guilds and Civil Society*, ch. 13.

8 David L. Cowen, 'Pharmacy and Freedom', *American Journal of Hospital Pharmacy*, 41 (1984), pp. 459–67.

9 N. McKendrick, J. Brewer, and J. H. Plumb, *The Birth of a Consumer Society* (London, 1982).

10 Roy Porter, *Disease, Medicine and Society in England 1550–1860* (Basingstoke, 1987), ch. 4.

11 S. W. F. Holloway, *Royal Pharmaceutical Society of Great Britain 1841–1991* (London, 1991), ch. 2.

12 This section is derived from: Logie Barrow, 'Democratic Epistemology: Mid-19th Century Plebian Medicine', *Society for the Social History of Medicine Bulletin*, 29 (1981), pp. 25–9; P. S. Brown, 'Herbalists and Medical Botanists in Mid-Nineteenth-Century Britain with Special Reference to Bristol', *Medical History*, 26 (1982), pp. 405–20; J. F. C. Harrison, 'Early Victorian Radicals and the Medical Fringe', in W. F. Bynum and Roy Porter, *Medical Fringe and Medical Orthodoxy 1750–1850* (London, 1987), pp. 198–215; Ursula Miley and John V. Pickstone, 'Medical Botany around 1850: American Medicine in

Industrial Britain', in Roger Cooter, ed., *Studies in the History of Alternative Medicine* (Basingstoke, 1988), pp. 139–54; and John V. Pickstone, 'Medical Botany (Self-Help Medicine in Victorian England)', *Manchester Literary and Philosophical Society, Memoirs and Proceedings*, 119 (1976–7), pp. 85–95.

13 T. H. Marshall, *Class, Citizenship, and Social Development* (New York, 1965), pp. 158–79.

14 Jonathon Porritt, *Seeing Green* (Oxford, 1984).

15 Jacob Bell, *Observations Addressed to the Chemists and Druggists of Great Britain on the Pharmaceutical Society* (1841), pp. 5–8.

16 *The Chemist*, 1 (1840), p. 2.

17 *Pharmaceutical Journal*, 2 (1842–3), p. 741.

18 *Ibid.*, 12 (1852–3), p. 369.

19 *Chemist and Druggist*, 3 (1862), pp. 79–80.

20 *Pharmaceutical Journal*, 4 (1844–5), p. 295.

21 *Ibid.*, p. 101; 2 (1842–3), p. 678; 3 (1843–4), p. 511.

22 *Hansard*, CXVIII (1851), 111–18.

23 *Ibid.*, CXIX (1852), 467–8.

24 *Pharmaceutical Journal*, 1 (1841–2), p. 4.

25 *Ibid.*, 3 (1843–4), pp. 509–10.

26 *Parliamentary Papers*, 1865 (78), I, p. 107.

27 *Report from the Select Committee of the House of Lords on the Sale of Poisons Bill*, 1857, Session II (294), XII.

28 *Pharmaceutical Journal*, 17 (1857–8), p. 443.

29 H. C. G. Matthew, *Gladstone 1809–1874* (Oxford, 1986), p. 169.

30 José Harris, 'Society and the State in Twentieth-Century Britain', in F. M. L. Thompson, ed., *The Cambridge Social History of Britain 1750–1950*, vol. III (Cambridge, 1990), ch. 2, pp. 63–117.

31 Matthew, *Gladstone*, p. 116.

32 John Stuart Mill, *On Liberty*, ed. S. Collini (Cambridge, 1989), p. 17.

33 *Ibid.*, pp. 96–7.

34 Peter Bartrip, 'A "Pennurth of Arsenic for Rat Poison": The Arsenic Act, 1851 and the Prevention of Secret Poisoning', *Medical History*, 36 (1992), pp. 53–69.

FIVE

DAS KAISERLICHE GESUNDHEITSAMT
(IMPERIAL HEALTH OFFICE) AND THE
CHEMICAL INDUSTRY IN GERMANY
DURING THE SECOND EMPIRE: PARTNERS
OR ADVERSARIES?

ERIKA HICKEL

BROADLY this contribution is concerned with drug regulation in
Germany during 1871–1914, in particular with the interaction of the
government and the chemical industry in this area. From its beginning
the German chemical industry was not a uniformly organized industrial branch. Since the 1850s and 1860s, it was possible to differentiate
between the heavy chemicals (primary) industry and the preparations
(processing) industry. Whereas the interest and problems of the first lay
in the production of soda, sulphuric acid, potash, and fertilizers (in
conjunction with the rising coal and steel industries), the second
pursued its own interests and as such was the first to come into contact
with governmental health institutions. This distinct attitude of the
preparations industry is further underlined by the founding of a body,
in 1877, called the Verein zur Wahrung der Interessen der chemischen
Industrie (Association for Safeguarding the Interests of the Chemical
Industry).[1]

Analysing the health policy of the Empire, our main interest will be
the preparations industry. Its products fall into two large groups, coal
tar chemicals and fine chemicals – both are closely connected with the
pharmacy. The pharmacists, in Germany traditionally having the
privilege of preparing medicines, developed also an interest in fine
chemicals. The mid-nineteenth-century industrialization brought forth
such firms emerging from pharmacists' shops as Schering, Riedel, and
Merck.[2] Since the 1880s the dye manufacturers began to develop
medicines from waste products or by-products. Some of the best-known
companies were Hoechst, Kalle, and Bayer.[3]

Historical writing gives prominence to the primary industry out of all
proportion although the big upturn in the chemical industry, between
1871 and 1914, took place mostly in the processing industry. Statistics
for this time-span of employment figures and exports corroborate this –

one of the reasons was a particularly favourable professional infrastructure.[4] At the beginning of the expansion period not only money for
investments (stemming from French reparations payments) was available but also potential specialist personnel. A number of former
apprentices, well trained in pharmacists' shops with laboratories
attached, moved to chemical institutes of universities for further education.[5] The majority of these university graduates found a place in the
chemical industry, and thus a close connection between university and
industry became established.[6] Through its close affinity with science the
German preparations industry could command already in the 1870s a
world-dominating position. At the same time, this situation required a
specific policy necessarily opposed to the demands of the Central Union
of German Industrialists (controlled by German heavy industry) for
special protective tariffs, in an endeavour to overcome foreign competition. The preparations industry, on the other hand, because of its
world-dominating position could be more 'liberal'; it was even in
favour of dismantling customs barriers. Therefore, the Association for
Safeguarding the Interests of the Chemical Industry opposed Bis-
marck's protectionist policy of 1879.[7]

By a few examples I can illustrate the basis of the worldwide preeminence of the German preparations industry. First, there were coal
tar dyes and fine chemicals which I do not wish to consider here, and
second, the synthetic medicinal chemicals. What I seek is to give a brief
treatment of some of the economic and scientific problems encountered
by the latter.[8]

Chloral hydrate was first manufactured in 1869. It was the first
synthetic sleep-inducing preparation on the market, not dependent on
natural products. This was the beginning of a series of experimental
investigations out of which preparations such as Sulfonal (1889) and
Veronal (1903) were derived. From the scientific point of view this
stimulated the endeavour to find connections between chemical
structure and pharmacological action.[9]

In 1873 Kolbe produced salicylic acid synthetically and thus for the
first time natural salicin was imitated for analgesic and antipyretic
purposes. This sparked off the famous dispute about patent rights
between Heyden and Schering, demonstrating the continuously
growing importance of patent and trademark legislation.[10] In connection with the marketing, by Kalle in 1886, of the chemically long-
known acetanilide as 'Antifebrine', it became apparent for the first time
that in the preparations industry protection of the trademark was far
more important than protection of the patent. It was often quite easy to
prepare a product by a different synthetic method and therefore the

trademark alone protected the product for the firm, at least for a few years.

Antipyrine shows several interesting aspects of drug manufacture. It was first produced by Hoechst in 1884 from phenylhydrazine, a starting material for the synthesis of yellow dyes, demonstrating the close connection between the production of drugs and dyes.[11] It is also a substitute for natural quinine. Another well-known development was Pyramidone. Phenacetine was discovered in 1886 and produced by Bayer on a large scale from 1887 onwards. It was derived from a by-product of coal tar dye manufacture (p-nitrophenol). This reveals a few basic principles in the chemical industry which still hold good today: use of by-products derived from other synthesis; quick exploitation of work in developmental stages, and close contact with pharmacology and clinical practice.[12]

The German preparations industry drew from its successes the self-confidence to promote its achievements by an almost modern public relations exercise. Thus already in 1884 Hoechst sent an extensive letter to Das Kaiserliche Gesundheitsamt (KGA) (Imperial Health Office) in which the benefits to the public of its working programme of pharmaceutical synthesis was expounded.[13] This indicated considerable foresight because at this time the significance of the authority of the KGA was still slight. Its establishment (1876) came at a time when the individual German states still found it hard to transfer their powers to central Imperial institutions. This meant that the KGA was only there in an advisory capacity, health administration and legislation was still in the hands of individual states.[14] The only legislative activity the KGA was allowed to pursue, since 1882, was the drawing up of the Imperial pharmacopoeia (Deutsches Arzneibuch – DAB).[15] In spite of the restrictions the KGA soon found a way to influence legislation in the individual states. It produced draft bills, which could be passed by the Federal Council (Bundesrat) and then sent on to the individual states for identical adoption.[16]

Many activities of the KGA are well known, for example, measures to combat epidemics, promotion of hygiene and microbiology, development of medical statistics. Other initiatives such as drug control, in which the KGA took a very early interest, are not known even to specialists. About this and about contacts with industry and universities more is to come.

There are several reasons why the activities with respect to the control of drugs by the KGA have hardly been noted. First, many of its initiatives in this direction did not come to fruition because the draft bills were not passed for reasons beyond the influence of the KGA.[17]

Second, the state of affairs with respect to source material is not encouraging enough to explore the subject. The KGA kept records from the start, but unfortunately they only partially survived the Second World War and are now with the Federal Archives at Koblenz. It appears that the first years after 1876 are only partially documented. For example, the revision of DAB between 1882 and 1900. This material is supplemented from the Imperial Chancellor's Office and also from the Prussian Ministry of Church, Education, and Medical Affairs, kept at Merseburg (especially the correspondence between the Imperial Authority (Reichsbehörde) and the Prussian Medical Department).

I had thought that the archives of some companies might hold records but, unfortunately, the most important firms have not been helpful. Schering and Merck have not responded to my queries.

To my knowledge the three most important areas with which the KGA wrestled between 1876 and 1914 were: first, quality control of medicinal chemicals; second, testing of the pharmaceutical industry's 'specialities' (patent medicines); third, control of galenical preparations. From the beginning the preparations industry paid attention to these questions, even though it does not appear to be so at first glance. There was the major problem that in German states traditionally the responsibility for drugs was handed down by the legislator to the pharmacist. But as the output of industrially produced pharmaceuticals grew this task was made more difficult because the analytical specifications were not provided quickly enough.

MEDICINAL CHEMICALS

When the KGA was set up in 1876, the purity of chemicals was already under discussion. Whereas in the last Prussian pharmacopoeia the choice of testing procedures was left to the pharmacists, the first German pharmacopoeia (1872) laid down certain specifications, although only a few, for the first time.[18]

A year later five of the main pharmaceutical firms (Schering, Merck, Gehe, Marquardt, and Trommsdorff) welcomed publicly this innovation.[19] Altogether they could do this safely because their preparations then in use complied with the requirements fully. The newly created KGA took this to be the right area to gain status. But either because of ignorance or in an effort to make itself distinct from its Prussian predecessor, the KGA first argued for the lowering of purity standards.[20] This appears to be incomprehensible in view of the already wide tolerance allowed in the first edition of DAB. A remarkable swing of opinion occurred, when the KGA, in 1878, started to work on its own pharmacopoeia for the first time – in effect the second edition of DAB (1882).

As newer and better methods of analysis were introduced, the discretionary powers of analysts were greatly curtailed. Newer methods included volumetric analysis and improved melting point determinations.[21] It should also be noted that specialists from inside and outside universities became members of the Pharmacopoeia Commission. Among them, the distinguished analyst Poleck was Professor of Pharmaceutical Chemistry in Breslau. Although industry was as yet not represented in the Pharmacopoeia Commission, this did not mean that it was without influence. Reber notes that the Commission members asked the manufacturer Schering 'on the quiet' for his opinion.[22] Schering demanded very high standards of purity, and he could do so because his firm was renowned for manufacturing and using purest chemicals (especially photographic chemicals).[23] In the eyes of competitors (probably Merck, Riedel, Boehringer, and perhaps Gehe and Trommsdorff) the second edition of DAB appeared to be too strict and they protested against it in a circular, the knowledge of which I have only at second hand.[24]

The KGA noted the complaints and then presumably passed them on to Poleck, who appointed his collaborator Thümmel at the University of Breslau to test the chemicals in common use by the method complained of. His conclusions were that most of the test procedures, prescribed by DAB, were appropriate; some were too tolerant and about one fifth were too strict.[25] That was the last time a university acted as an independent arbitrator between the KGA and industry.

When the third edition of DAB was being prepared, the Schering partner J. F. Holtz, could influence the setting of purity standards.[26] What influence he had can only be guessed; the fact is that the third edition set even higher purity standards.[27] That these standards favoured Schering against its less efficient and possibly cheaper competitors can not be easily refuted. On the Pharmacopoeia Commission for the fourth edition of DAB (1900) Holtz was no longer alone in setting the tone. He was joined by another representative of the industry, the highly enterprising Louis Merck. What influence he brought to bear on the setting of test specifications we do not know, as the relevant papers are missing. We can only inspect the fourth edition of DAB from this point and note that the purity standards were not raised – on the contrary they were partially lowered again. A great many 'pure' reagents were included – mainly manufactured, as it happens, by Merck Co.

In contrast the influence of the industry on testing procedures incorporated into the fifth edition of DAB can be proven, as the relevant records have been preserved.[28] The tests for chemicals in this pharmacopoeia were drawn up by Merck himself; the Professor of Pharmaceutical Chemistry Beckurts acted as the second expert but I do not know how well these two agreed with one another.

If a historian desires to judge the described developments, he has to remember the actual purpose of a pharmacopoeia. It was and is to provide the medical man and the pharmacist, and so indirectly the patient, with a state-controlled authoritative standard of quality for medicinal drugs. The actual development violated this intention. The KGA and the university professors lost, as we have seen, more and more their role of control authorities to the inevitably commercially orientated industry.

However, what should not be overlooked is that there are two sides to the purity requirement of medicinal drugs. On the one hand, it caused the manufacturers to exert themselves to improve their production processes without necessarily affecting the price of the product.[29] On the other hand, the price of drugs could rise disproportionately through higher costs of production. As no one knew with certainty the limit of the physiologically damaging effect of impurities, the standards for purity were set very high. Without a countercheck it was possible for the representatives of the industry to manipulate the purity criteria in order to maximize their profit margins.

PROPRIETARY MEDICINES ('SPECIALITIES')

As already mentioned, the KGA had a second problem to deal with, i.e. the control of specialities or proprietary drugs. In 1870 there were only a few dozen proprietary medicines ready packed in the factory and mostly protected by trademarks – by 1914 their number was more than 10,000.[30] The explosive increase should have reminded the KGA that it was its task to prepare necessary legislative measures. Moreover, it became apparent that there were attempts to make easy money by marketing medicines whose ingredients were secret, or even fraudulent preparations.

As the economy expanded, the number of drug manufacturers grew drastically and the market was flooded with synthetic drugs. As already mentioned, medicinal substances were provided with officially registered trademarks. This led newcomers to market the same substance under another name or alleged chemical derivatives as proprietary medicines. The supply was even more increased by making use of all possible combinations of these substances in preparations, including some already obsolete medicines. In part the criminal threshold was already crossed with so-called 'secret preparations'. What it actually meant was that their composition was not declared, which was legal at that time. Clearly, some manufacturers advertising their products endowed them with imaginary ingredients and properties.[31] The boom on the drug market was enhanced, as pointed out by Vershofen, in 1889 by setting up the general health insurance scheme, which made more money available for the provision of medicines.

The fraudulent practices of the drug market were later blamed on the so-called 'scullery firms' (*Waschküchenfirmen*), but the big firms knew how to cash in on the economic boom through a few tricks of their own. Thus Hoechst marketed Antipyrine under four different brand names with widely differing prices. As their competitor Louis Merck later ascertained, all four preparations were identical in composition if not in price.[32] When the third edition of DAB was being prepared (1890), the question of proprietary preparations appeared to the KGA of little import. The main concern was to classify the new synthetic drugs either as non-toxic (*indifferent*) or poisonous (*giftig*). By submitting clinical reports the manufacturers tried to substantiate their harmlessness.[33] However, the KGA eventually came to the opposite conclusion on the basis of looking through foreign specialist journals.[34] This was the first indication that the KGA was adopting a critical attitude towards the preparations industry. The deplorable state of affairs in the drug market could no longer be overlooked.[35]

Besides, several organizations representing pharmacists and physicians respectively complained to the authorities[36] and thus provoked the KGA into drawing up a statutory regulation regarding secret remedies that was issued by the Federal Council (Bundesrat) in 1903. The physicians and pharmacists felt immediately that the regulation was inadequate. Thus the Prussian Chambers of Pharmacy demanded from the KGA the grading of all new proprietary medicines and remedies with secret ingredients, either a non-toxic or strongly effective (*starkwirksam*).[37] Their argument was that the statute of 1903 presented only a negative register of forbidden preparations which became almost immediately out of date. The KGA did not comply with these demands on account of the expense involved in conducting necessary pharmacological and clinical tests. Pharmacists and physicians were consoled with a promise of a supplement to the statutory regulation for 1907 affecting medicines with secret ingredients. This was to contain not only a list of unauthorized medicines with secret ingredients but also the prohibition of false descriptions of the contents on drug packages.

The university professors His and Thoms, in their capacity as chairmen of important associations (German Society for Combating Quackery: German Pharmaceutical Society), pointed to the inadequacy of the new Act already in 1908.[38] They were right to criticize inasmuch as the negative list could not stop the flooding of the market with ever more medicines containing secret ingredients. They also campaigned against the fact that the composition of proprietary drugs had still not to be declared. Moreover, they denounced the still allowed bad custom of advertising false claims in specialized periodicals which went unpunished. Some pharmacists and institutes of pharmaceutical chemistry tried to throw some light on the composition of the preparations,[39] but they were overwhelmed by the flood of products and could not cope with it.[40] His and Thoms demanded the setting up of a central institution for the testing of drugs, which seemed the right thing to do. A preparatory committee, consisting of interested pharmaceutical and medical university teachers and representatives of Bayer Co., met on 28 June 1908.[41] It specified again the well-known demands and asked the KGA for support. The planned central institution was to create conditions for analysing all marketed proprietary drugs in order to eliminate fraudulent declarations. In a statement the KGA welcomed the plan but thought it unworkable. Apart from legal complications, the KGA feared that the anger of the industry could erupt into legal actions and claims for damages against the analysts. Without a 'Drugs Act' to fall back on, the KGA believed that it could not succeed against the industry–state partnership, committed to freedom of trade (*Gewerbefreiheit*). Remarkably, the KGA perceived the necessity of having such a law.[42] Taking stock of the attitude of the KGA with respect to proprietary drugs, it has to be said that it possessed foresight but lacked persuasive drive. However, here one must take into consideration that the extent of outside influences, on the basis of extant papers, can not be fully assessed.

GALENICALS

The third and last problem the KGA had to tackle was quite different. There is so much source material which confirms the massive influence upon the KGA beyond a shadow of doubt. One cannot be but impressed how skilfully the industrial lobby proceeded at that time. Superficially, the production and control of galenicals respectively did not seem to justify the considerable expenditure on writing material for petitions but interested parties quickly realized that a case of precedence was involved. Common opinion had it that galenicals such as ointments, plasters, plant extracts (tinctures and essences) were not suitable for analytical testing and their preparation was left *de iure* in the hands of pharmacists even after 1871. It was believed that this provided the sole guarantee for the right constitution and quality of these items.[43] Doubtless then galenicals played a far greater role than today.[44]

Already since the beginning of the nineteenth century a 'grey' area existed in the galenicals market. As already mentioned, only the pharmacists had the right to make them up. But the industry was offering these products and was also finding buyers among pharmacists.[45] After 1900 this market grew so rapidly that the KGA found it necessary to clarify the situation. A powerful impetus to deal with it was given when the KGA, in 1905, drew up the official scale of retail charges for medicines (*Arzneitaxe*) for the first time. At the same time, it became evident that the price for galenicals set by the industrial producers were differing widely and also that this business greatly expanded.

At first internally, the KGA drafted a bill restating the obligation of pharmacists to be responsible for the preparation of most galenicals.[46] The old arguments were used. That is, in many German states it was anyhow obligatory for the pharmacists to prepare galenicals, and the official scale of retail charges for them was calculated on this basis. Further, only in this way could their proper constitution and quality be ensured.[47] Early in 1909 the KGA communicated its intentions regarding the bill in specialist journals. Protests from industrialists followed immediately. To widen the basis for discussion the KGA called a conference with experts from the Imperial Health Council. This was an honorary advisory body attached to the KGA since 1901, consisting of scientific, industrial, and professional experts and bureaucrats. Apparently, the KGA tried to restrict the size of the conference because Louis Merck, a member of the advisory body, was not invited at first. After protesting through telephone calls and telegrams he obtained an invitation in the end but the KGA invited eight other big industrialists and a representative from the small-scale industry, possibly for reasons of parity.[48]

The industry tried to use the time between January and May, the publishing date of the draft bill, to its advantage. It organized an orchestrated and escalating wave of protest letters addressed to the KGA and Federal Council.[49] It began with a letter from Merck Co. protesting, in general terms, against the exclusion of the industry from consultations. The arguments of the industry were then set out, in particular, in a letter from Riedel Co. to the KGA. First, the industrial manufacture of galenicals gave work to 15,000 blue-collar and 5,000 white-collar workers;[50] second, only the industry backed up by its scientific expertise could guarantee the consistent quality of galenicals[51] (the implication being that pharmacists could not);[52] third, centralization of the production of galenicals in large pharmacies was not to be welcomed, it would lead to the formation of a new industry;[53] fourth, pharmacy-made preparation (*Selbstherstellung*) necessarily increases the scale of charges;[54] fifth, the export business of German firms would be impeded;[55] sixth, in case of mobilization pharmacies would not have sufficient stocks.[56]

We can see that the industry was not too fussy in putting forward reasons in support of its case by bringing in science, nationalism, altruism, and even bogus contentions. The same company (Riedel) also addressed the Federal Council, which was responsible for legislation, with the aim of damaging the reputation of pharmacists and presenting the industrial performance to its best advantage. The crux of the argument in the letter was the assertion that whereas the hitherto governmental support of the industry was a sign of 'movement and progress', the initiative of the KGA was 'a step backwards'.

In February 1909 the Association of Medicinal Drug Traders – to which Riedel, among others, belonged – became active. It also employed the two-pronged route of soliciting both the KGA and the Federal Council. Apart from the already known arguments, the letters contained the following additional points: with the present practice (viz. 'grey market') no grievances had come to light; the industrially manufactured medicines were 'better' than those prepared in pharmacies;[57] the KGA had ignored the transition from pharmacies into industrial establishments during the last fifty to seventy-five years, and therefore was 'retrograde and obscurantist'.

The apex of this campaign was a memorandum submitted by the Association for Safeguarding the Interests of the Chemical Industry, in February 1909, in which the already massive argumentation was strengthened by threats: the state would be liable to pay compensation for losses sustained arising out of the enactment. The organization applied not only the stick but also offered a carrot. Accordingly, the industry was prepared to employ sworn pharmacists and submit to annual auditing, as commonly practised in pharmacies.[58]

The question has to be asked what it was that made the industry go to such lengths. The precedental nature of the affair was already referred to. Ultimately it concerned the question who was to be responsible for medicines in the future, especially for the trade in tablets. Although during this period the sale of tablets developed into big business, their preparation in Germany was by law still a pharmacist prerogative. If the industry was permitted to manufacture galenicals, the door to industrial production of proprietary tablets would also be opened. In fact the Association began in 1909 its campaign to be allowed to deliver tablets also to wholesalers. This depended on granting the industry the right to test drugs itself.[59]

In the conference convened by the KGA all the arguments of the industry and the counter-arguments of the KGA came to the fore.[60] After the scientists, professional representatives and health officials rejected the industry's arguments as not valid, it came to the vote. There was only one dissenter, namely Louis Merck, the sole representative of the industry.[61]

In May 1910 the KGA sent a final report regarding galenicals to the Ministry of the Interior.[62] It once more underlined the reasons for the exclusive right of pharmacists to prepare galenicals, unless the economic interests of the industry spoke against them. This counter-argument prevailed and the draft never became law. With this the industry took over the responsibility for drug control, creating problems for the future which are not for discussion here.

What then was the attitude of the KGA to the industry during the Second Empire? Was it a partner or was it an adversary? It has to be said that it was both. At the beginning the KGA was inclined to help industry. Later, during industry's growth, it became wary especially in the face of apparent failings. Certainly lower rank officials did not always see eye to eye with those who presided over the KGA. While the former could remain objective, the latter had to take political interests into consideration. They had to bow to the 'higher' viewpoints of the state government, which in this instance meant to take on board the economic and political power of the industry.

NOTES

This is the English version – slightly abridged and revised – of the article originally published in German 'Das Kaiserliche Gesundheitsamt und die chemische Industrie im Zweiten Kaiserreich (1871–1914): Partner oder Kontrahenten?', in G. Mann and R. Winau, eds., *Medizin, Naturwissenschaft, Technik und das Zweite Kaiserreich* (Göttingen, 1977), pp. 64–86.

1 For a contemporary, still useful historical account, see H. Schulze, *Die Entwicklung der chemischen Industrie in Deutschland seit dem Jahre 1875. Eine volkswirtschaftliche Studie* (Halle/S., 1908). Here all branches of the chemical industry are dealt with.

2 G. Urdang, 'Die deutsche Apotheke als Keimzelle der deutschen pharmazeutischen Industrie', in *Die Vorträge der Hauptversammlung in Wien (= Veröffentlichungen der Deutschen Gesellschaft für Geschichte der Pharmazie)* (Mittenwald, n.d., [1931]), pp. 93–153.

3 A. J. Ihde, *The Development of Modern Chemistry* (New York, 1964), pp. 443–71,

671–94; W. Schneider, *Geschichte der pharmazeutischen Chemie* (Weinheim, 1972), pp. 279–304.

4 Schulze, *Entwicklung*, pp. 16, 32ff, 96ff, 104ff, 180ff, 191–4; *Die chemische Industrie* 32 (1909), p. 37; W. G. Hoffmann, *Das Wachstum der deutschen Wirtschaft seit der Mitte des 19. Jahrhunderts* (Berlin, 1965), p. 196; W. Rudolph, 'Die Wechselwirkungen zwischen den chemischen Instituten der Technischen Hochschule Dresden und der Industrie im Zeitraum von 1870 bis 1900' (Dissertation, Dresden, 1970), vol. II, p. 138.

5 Thus most of Liebig's students at Giessen came originally from pharmacists' shops. Significantly, during Liebig's lifetime, the journal he published went under the name *Annalen der Pharmazie* (1832–9) and *Annalen der Pharmazie und Chemie* (1840–73) respectively.

6 Cf. J. S. Fruton on Adolf von Baeyer's research school and the German chemical industry in *Contrasts in Scientific Style Research Groups in the Chemical and Biochemical Sciences* (Philadelphia, 1990), pp. 158ff; O. Krätz, *Beilstein – Erlenmeyer. Briefe* (Munich, 1972); *idem*, 'Der Chemiker in den Gründerjahren', in E. Schmauderer, ed., *De Chemiker im Wandel der Zeiten* (Weinheim, 1973), pp. 259–84.

7 Cf. the issues of *Die chemische Industrie* since 1878; W. Vershofen, *Wirtschaftsgeschichte der chemisch-pharmazeutischen Industrie*, vol. III: 1870–1914 (Aulendorf, 1958). For another partial aspect of the history of the Association, see R. Sonnemann, 'Der Einfluss des Patentwesens auf die Herausbildung von Monopolen in der deutschen Teerfarbenindustrie (1877–1914) (Habilitation Thesis, University of Halle-Wittenberg, 1963), pp. 158–88. Some members of the Association later became members of the KGA, for example, J. F. Holtz (Schering Co.) and Louis Merck. On the influence of interest groups on politics in the Imperial age see W. Fischer, 'Staatsverwaltung und Interessenverbände im Deutschen Reich 1871–1914', in C. Böhret and D. Grosser, eds., *Interdependenzen von Politik und Wirtschaft. Festgabe für Gerd v. Eynern* (Berlin, 1967), pp. 431–56.

8 See Vershofen, *Wirtschaftsgeschichte*; Ihde, *Development*: Schneider, *Geschichte*. There are many more examples also in P. Siedler, *Die chemischen Arzneimittel der letzten 113 Jahre* (Berlin, 1914).

9 B. Issekutz, *Die Geschichte der Arzneimittelforschung* (Budapest, 1971), p. 77.

10 The Imperial Patent Law which protected the method of preparation of substances dates from 1876, the trademark legislation from 1894.

11 As a further development of the quinine substitute Kairine.

12 Thus the medical professors Kast, Bäumler, Gerhardt, and Friedrich Müller worked for Bayer and Mehring and Kobert for Merck in the 1880s, Federal Archives Koblenz, R-86, No. 1654 and 1642; *Mercks Berichte* (1888), p. 30.

13 Among other things this was done in order to prevent the classification of the new Antipyrine as a preparation available in pharmacies only. In translation the relevant passage reads as follows: 'The intermediary role of the [pharmacy] is a thorough hindrance. Let it be allowed, for example, to discuss the Antipyrine trade. We were concerned to get the Antipyrine as cheap as possible to the sick. We thought that this could be best achieved by taking the risk for the new remedy at the outset that a pharmacist (*Apotheker*) or a druggist (*Droguist*) has to take anyhow. We did this by undertaking the obligation with respect to the

druggists directly and with respect to the pharmacists indirectly, to take back all unopened tins (25 g) at any time. We sell Antipyrine to druggists at 96 Marks per kg (M120,- with a discount of 20%), to pharmacies on urgent request at M120,-, and to hospital pharmacists at M108,-. Taking the prices into account, our profit may be approximately calculated realizing that two of the raw materials for the manufacture of Antipyrine, that is phenylhydrazine and acetoaceticester, are hitherto not produced on a large scale [and hence are] expensive. It could then be expected that the pharmacist bought Antipyrine at M120,- per kg and sold it at M200,- per kg or 20 Pfennig per g. But he sells Antipyrine at a much higher price and therefore discredits it with the physician. If it is to one's credit to have discovered a medically valuable substance, and further if a chemical factory can claim the merit to produce it on a large scale, then what credit goes to the individual pharmacist [in this matter]? He cannot possibly guarantee the purity of the substance because he does not know its properties' (the properties of Antipyrine were described in the third edition DAB (1891)). See Federal Archives Koblenz, R-86 (*Reichsgesundheitsamt*), No. 1642. Letter of Farbwerke vorm. Meister, Lucius and Brüning, Hoechst/ M., 12 July 1884, fols. 51v–52r.

14 On the history of the KGA, see *Das Reichsgesundheitsamt 1876–1926. Festschrift hrsg. vom Reichsgesundheitsamt aus Anlass seines fünfzigjährigen Bestehens* (Berlin, 1926); O. Rapmund, *Das öffentliche Gesundheitswesen* (Leipzig, 1901), pp. 62–5, 135–7.

15 Its forerunners were composed by the authorities in the individual states: for example, the Prussian pharmacopoeia by the Technical Commission for Pharmaceutical Affairs at the Ministry of Church, Education, and Medical Affairs (Kultusministerium) in Berlin. Cf. E. Hickel, 'Arzneimittelkommissionen bei der Preussischen Regierung 1798–1862', *Rete – Strukturgeschichte der Naturwissenschaften*, 2 (1974), pp. 143–67. The first edition of DAB (1872) was produced by the Technical Commission set up by the Federal Council (Bundesrat); cf. W. Schneider, 'Vorgeschichte der ersten Pharmacopoea Germanica', *Pharmazeutische Zeitung*, 104 (1959), pp. 495–9, 519ff, 1985–90. After 1876 the Technical Commission as well as the newly founded KGA tried to compile a new edition of the German pharmacopoeia. After some controversy, the KGA appointed the Commission in 1878. German Central Archives Merseburg, Rep. 76 VIII A, No. 1761.

16 There was no comprehensive Drug Control Act before 1961. Between 1871 and 1914 the drug trade was controlled at the individual state level and at the Empire level respectively by several ordinances and laws.

17 The KGA was neither a legislative nor an administrative body – it was merely an advisory institution. As such, it was entitled to draft bills and ordinances and submit them to the Imperial Chancellor's Office (Reichskanzleramt).

18 E. Hickel, *Arzneimittel-Standardisierung in den Pharmakopöen des 19. Jahrhunderts in Deutschland, Frankreich, Grossbritannien und den Vereinigten Staaten von America* (Stuttgart, 1973), pp. 75–84, 91–8; *idem*, 'Die Pharmakopöe, ein Spiegel ihrer Zeit (Tschirch.)', *Medizinhistorisches Journal* 6 (1971), 207–12; *idem*, 'Probleme bei der Einführung chemisch-analytischer Prüfmethoden in die Pharmakopöen', *Veröffentlichungen der Gesellschaft für Geschichte der Pharmazie*, n.s., 38 (1972), pp. 165–71; *idem*, 'Hundert Jahre Deutsches Arzneibuch', *Pharmazeutische Industrie*, 34 (1972), pp. 581–3.

19 German Central Archives Merseburg, Rep. 76 VIII A, No. 1761, fol. 150v.

20 *Ibid.*, 150r.

21 Hickel,   *Arzneimittel-Standardisierung*,   pp. 13,   75–84,   92–8,   142–9;   *idem*,
    'Probleme'.

22 B. Reber, *Gallerie [sic] hervorragender Therapeutiker und Pharmakognosten der Gegen-
    wart* (Geneva, 1897), pp. 376–8.

23 *Ibid.*, 376; Schulze, *Entwicklung*, pp. 93ff.

24 Which chemical firms are meant in this circular one can only guess because the
    relevant papers of the KGA are missing, cf. Vershofen, *Wirtschaftsgeschichte*. See
    also W. Bernsmann, 'Arzneimittelforschung und -entwicklung in Deutschland
    in der zweiten Hälfte des 19. Jahrhunderts', *Die pharmazeutische Industrie*, 29
    (1967), pp. 448ff, 525–9, 669–73, 745–8, 834–6, 963–6, 1032–5, and 30 (1968),
    pp. 58–9, 131–2, 199, 342–4, 408–9, 471–3; J. H. Merck, *Entwicklung und Stand
    der pharmazeutischen Gross-Industrie Deutschlands* (Berlin, 1923), p. 50; *Die chemische
    Industrie*, 1 (1878), pp. 1–3; Federal Archives Koblenz, R-86, Nos. 1530 and
    1533.

25 K. Thümmel, 'Zur Kritik der Prüfungsmethoden der Pharmac. Germ. ed. II',
    Archiv der Pharmazie, 222 (1884), pp. 793–822.

26 Reber, *Gallerie*; H. Schelenz, *Geschichte der Pharmazie* (Berlin, 1904), pp. 770.
    J. F. Holtz was a founder member of the Association for Safeguarding of the
    Interests of the Chemical Industry. He was an old friend of E. Schering and was
    also friendly with the Russian pharmacist and author of the Russian pharmaco-
    poeia v. Trapp. Reber (in *Gallerie*) writes that 'Holtz had not an insignificant
    influence on the purity standards laid down in the Russian pharmacopoeia
    [1891]. He was naturally concerned that they met the standards of Schering's
    preparations. In this he was successful also from the material point of view.' J. F.
    Holtz became a member of the permanent Pharmacopeia Commission in 1892.

27 Hickel, *Arzneimittel-Standardisierung*, pp. 82, 92–4.

28 Federal Archives Koblenz, R-86, No. 1533, Vol. 1: 'Liste der zur Aufnahme in
    das Arzneibuch für das Deutsche Reich, fünfte Ausgabe, vorgesehenen Arznei-
    mittel nebst Angabe der Referenten'. Certain preparations containing second-
    ary plant principles were dealt with by E. Schmidt (Marburg) and Louis
    Merck. According to the list 'reagents for medico-chemical investigation' should
    have been originally worked on by v. Krehl, Weintraud and Binz, but, in fact,
    Louis Merck took over most of the drawing up of procedures. See notes in
    Federal Archives Koblenz, R-86, No. 1533, Vols. 1 and 2. The decisive influ-
    ence of the big firms led to protests by smaller manufacturers because they felt
    they were disadvantaged. Cf. their joint letter addressed to the KGA, Federal
    Archives Koblenz, R-86, No. 1533, May 1911.

29 Hickel, *Arzneimittel-Standardisierung*, pp. 93ff; E. Hickel, 'Die Pharmakopöe, ein
    Apothekerbuch?', *Pharmazie unserer Zeit*, 2 (1973), pp. 1–8.

30 E. Ernst tried to obtain a more exact definition of the specialities ('secret
    industrial preparations', 'pharmaceutical specialities', 'medicinal specialities'),
    a discussion of which goes beyond the scope of this article. Cf. his 'Das
    "industrielle" Geheimmittel und seine Werbung' (Dissertation, Marburg,
    1969). The KGA was of the opinion that the boundary between specialities and
    secret preparations should not be drawn too rigidly. See Report of the KGA to
    the Ministry of Interior, 23 October 1908, Federal Archives Koblenz, R-86,

No. 1585, Vol. 6. Ernst is to be credited with proving that advertisements played a big part in the speciality market even before 1914.

31 A typical case was the so-called pyrenol affair. The manufacturer gave the product a name and a new chemical formula although it was a 'melt' of long-known, common-place, chemicals. Cf. H. Thoms, 'Arzneimittelfabriktion in alter und neuer Zeit', *Berichte der deutschen pharmazeutischen Gesellschaft*, 18 (1909), pp. 369–93.

32 Louis Merck wrote on the subject during the preparation of the fourth edition of DAB (1910): 'The action of the Hoechst Co. serves without doubt their endeavour to induce pharmacists to purchase an expensive preparation, and thus underlines how questionable it is to label medicinal preparations with trademarks.' Federal Archives Koblenz, R-86, No. 1642, letters of 4 and 17 May 1900 to the KGA.

33 See n. 12. In 1896 at the Annual Meeting of German Physicians a resolution was passed for the first time against 'the misuse [by manufacturers as sales gimmick] of medical reports'.

34 Federal Archives Koblenz, R-86, No. 1654: 'Zusammenstellung der aus der Gesammt-Literatur bis zum Ende des Jahres 1889 entnommenen Notizen über die toxischen Wirkungen (*Nebenwirkungen*) des Antipyrin und Phenacetin'.

35 The KGA became even more aware of the abuses (see n. 32) when it began to look into the question of official drug prices (*Arzneitaxe*) in 1902, brought in in 1905. Hitherto this had been a matter for individual states.

36 For example, submission of the German Pharmacists' Association to the KGA (29 November 1900); submission of the Committee of the Prussian Chambers of Pharmacists to the Prussian Minister of Church, Education, and Medical Affairs (15 October 1903); submission of the German Society for Combating Quackery to the KGA (4 July 1905). Cf. Ernst, 'Geheimmittel', pp. 186–96.

37 This had a bearing on over-the-counter medicine sales be it inside or outside the pharmacy (according to the so-called Imperial Ordinance of 1901), but also on the sales of prescription medicines (according to the Apothecaries' Statute). Cf. also U. Meinecke, 'Apothekenbindung und Freiverkäuflichkeit von Arzneimitteln' (Dissertation, Marburg, 1972), pp. 203–7.

38 Federal Archives Koblenz, R-86, No. 1585, Vol. 6; Thoms, 'Arzneimittelfabrikation'.

39 Above all the pharmaceutical-chemical institutes of the university in Berlin (Thoms) and Breslau (Gadamer) and numerous pharmacists, cf. publications in the *Apotheker-Zeitung*. See also R. Schmitz, *Die deutschen pharmazeutisch-chemischen Hochschulinstitute* (Ingelheim, 1969), pp. 38–43, 83–6.

40 In 1908 public health officers regarded the publication of analytical findings in popular journals such as *Gartenlaube* as the only possible and effective way to counter the proprietary drugs deception. Cf. O. Rapmund, ed., *Das preussische Medizinal- und Gesundheitswesen in den Jahren 1883–1908. Festschrift zur Feier des 25 jährigen Bestehen des Prussischen Medizinalbeamten-Vereins* (Berlin, 1908), p. 463.

41 The meeting was attended by Eichengrün (Elberfeld), Heffter, His, Kutner, G. Lennhof (all from Berlin), Lomnitz (Elberfeld), Schwalbe (Berlin), Thoms (Steglitz). Federal Archives Koblenz, R-86, No. 1585, Vol. 6.

42 See Report cited in n. 30.

43 Cf. E. Hickel, 'Die Auseinandersetzung deutscher Apotheker mit Problemen

der Industrialisierung im 19. Jahrhundert', *Pharmazeutische-Zeitung*, 118 (1973), pp. 1635–44, 119 (1974), pp. 143–67, 1837–58. On galenicals, see Schneider, *Geschichte*, pp. 281ff; Hickel, *Arzneimittel-Standardisierung*, pp. 116ff, 157ff.

44 It is noteworthy that although the contemporary pharmacopoeia contains few directions regarding galenicals, their share in what the pharmacy has to offer is still respectable. There are hundreds of such articles for sale.

45 After 1875 more and more pharmacists, interpreting the legal situation to their advantage, purchased from wholesalers. This actually was contrary to the opinion of the KGA. See also Federal Archives Koblenz, R-86, No. 1585, Vol. 1 (copies 'Für die Registratur des Kaiserl. Gesundheitsamtes' March 1879). Cf. also Meinecke, 'Apothekenbindfung'.

46 Some galenical preparations which were unquestionably better produced industrially on a large scale were excluded from the start, such as Unguentum Hydrargyri nigrum. In August 1907 Holtz and Merck, as representatives of the KGA, were invited to attend the first consultations. Only Holtz participated but Merck later complained about the lack of information.

47 Federal Archives Koblenz, R-86, No. 1585, Vol. 6.

48 The large-scale industry was represented by Röttgen (Riedel, Berlin), Bausch (Gehe, Dresden), C. Dieterich (Helfenberg), P. Riedel, Köbner (Boehringer, Mannheim), Brunnengräber (Rostock), Witte (Rostock), and the representative of the Association for Safeguarding the Interests of the Chemical Industry. The divergent thinking of the small-scale industry (according to L. Merck) was represented by Evers (Reisholz near Düsseldorf). Federal Archives Koblenz, R-86, No. 1585, Vol. 7.

49 Federal Archives Koblenz, R-86, No. 1585, Vol. 7 – here also the counter-arguments of the KGA.

50 The figures were disputed by the KGA.

51 The pharmacists at the galenicals conference (19 May 1909) – especially Professor Beckurts – pointed out that the concentration of extracts, supplied by different firms, differed widely even though they carried the same name. KGA officials (Anselmino, Schmidt, Kerp) refuted the firms' claim that their testing methods, applied to galenicals, were accurate enough.

52 According to the KGA the Pharmacists' Ordinances ensured that they were sufficiently qualified to carry out the preparations of galenicals themselves.

53 The intention behind the bill of the KGA was to push for excluding centralization.

54 According to the KGA this was not correct, as the existing charges already took preparation in the pharmacy shop into account.

55 Although repeatedly requested by the KGA, the representatives of the industry were never prepared to disclose export figures of galenicals.

56 This was disputed by the representative of the military *Oberstabsapotheker* Devin at the conference on 19 May 1909.

57 Some medicines supplied by the industry were stronger because they were not prepared according to specifications laid down in the pharmacopoeia. This was condemned by the medical expert (Kraus) present at the meeting on 19 May 1909 because clinical experience and therapeutic practice were based on DAB criteria. This was especially true for extracts and tinctures which had to be prepared, according to the DAB, by maceration but were industrially often

produced by percolation. This latter procedure made them clearer and mostly better coloured but also often stronger and therefore more dangerous.

58 The KGA regarded this in the nature of a lip-service offer because such a control could not be carried out on account of the freedom of trade.

59 C. A. v. Martius' 'Reform der Gesetzgebung betreffend die zusammengepressten Arzneizubereitungen', *Die chemische Industrie*, 32 (1909), pp. 33–4.

60 Federal Archives Koblenz, R-86, No. 1585, Vol. 7. Minutes of the meeting on 19 May 1909 and Final Report of the KGA (prepared by Schmidt and Kerp) sent to the Minister of the Interior on 25 May 1910.

61 Entitled to vote were members of the Imperial Health Council Beckurts and Paul (Professors of Pharmacy), Kraus (Professor of Medicine), pharmacists (Salzmann and Schweissinger) the industrialist Louis Merck and several medical officials. Conspicuously absent from the meeting on 19 May 1909 were other members of the Imperial Health Council, that is Professors A. Meyer and E. Schmidt, the pharmacists V. Pieverling, Brunnengräber and Witte (the latter two were invited as representatives of industry).

62 In time for the draft to take effect simultaneously with the publication of the 5th edition of DAB (1 January 1911).

SIX

FROM ALL PURPOSE ANODYNE TO MARKER OF DEVIANCE: PHYSICIANS' ATTITUDES TOWARDS OPIATES IN THE US FROM 1890 TO 1940

CAROLINE JEAN ACKER

ALTHOUGH opiates are among the oldest medicines known to humankind, they continue to spark new discoveries in the workings of the brain. And although they remain of interest at the cutting edge of pharmacological research, opiates continue to be mired in intractable social problems. This essay examines the attitudes of physicians toward opiates from about 1890 to 1940. As part of the larger effort to transform medicine into a powerful and self-regulating profession in this period, American physicians sought to increase their control over the distribution of medicines to the sick. In the late nineteenth century, the harm associated with the unregulated American drug market provoked reformers both within and without the profession to action. Opiates were a target of concern because of their prevalence in proprietary medicines, their centrality in therapeutics, their association with symptom-relieving rather than curative medicine, and the risk they posed for addiction. To gauge these concerns, I will examine two kinds of sources. First, charting the actions of the American Medical Association (AMA) shows the role of opiates in the public effort to transform medicine and shake off charges of iatrogenic addiction. Second, within the profession, more private concerns about opiates in medical practice can be traced by surveying textbooks and manuals of materia medica and therapeutics.

OPIATES IN THE PUBLIC ARENA

By 1900, the foundations for a new explanatory basis for medicine had been developed. These included the elucidation of bacterial causes of such diseases as tuberculosis, and the development of immunization procedures to prevent some diseases and of sera to treat others. Physicians and public health workers had powerful new tools to fight disease, tools which increased the authority of these two groups to mandate social changes in the name of health.[1]

Medical education was reformed along the lines of the German laboratory-based teaching to improve the quality of medical practice and eliminate substandard schools.[2] Although reform initiatives had been underway from the 1870s,[3] substantial institutional reorganization occurred after 1900. The AMA reorganized in 1901 and undertook wide-ranging and vigorous activities in public education and lobbying in the interest of the private practitioner.[4]

With respect to drugs, three objectives can be discerned in the actions of the AMA. One was to transform therapeutics along modern, scientific lines. A second goal was to increase medical control over who took what drugs. This was to be achieved not through overt economic control of the market place, but through bolstering the physician's authority to determine what drugs were useful in what conditions. Finally, the prescribing practices of careless or mercenary physicians must be curbed. Opiates were central to all three areas of concern.

Scientific findings of the late nineteenth century led many physicians to challenge traditional explanations of disease and hope for the advent of more effective remedies than those already known. New methods of drug development, pioneered in Germany, offered the promise of drugs which could attack the causes of individual diseases.[5] Paul Ehrlich's Salvarsan, a new treatment for syphilis developed from a form of arsenic, was described in conceptual terms as a magic bullet, a drug which performed a single, specific, targeted action.

The impact of new disease explanations and new drug possibilities was spelled out in a 1915 report of the AMA's Council on Pharmacy and Chemistry. This body had been created in 1905 to discredit purveyors of harmful or useless medicines and to test and approve useful new drugs.[6] 'Forty years ago', wrote the report's authors, 'the conditions of medical practice were essentially the same as at the time of Sydenham. We possessed a few great therapeutic agents whose use had been learned empirically . . . There was little recognition . . . of the true nature of disease.'[7] One hallmark of the old-fashioned therapeutics was the application of the same medicine for a wide-ranging list of indications. Indeed, for many poorly understood conditions, 'pretty much everything in the Pharmacopoeia could with advantage be employed'.[8] Salvarsan exemplified the new therapeutics, but unfortunately, there were as yet few remedies which could effectively strike diseases at their cause. Continued progress would be arduous, as 'Ehrlich seems to have had at least 605 failures before approaching his goal',[9] but improving education in and laboratory facilities for pharmacology was expected to hasten the advent of new medicines. An important function of the Council was to test newly developed medications.

Those it approved of were listed annually in *New and Nonofficial Remedies*, a series of volumes to make promising new drugs known to practitioners before they had been included in the US pharmacopoeia.

The AMA's faith in drug development was based on almost a century's work, beginning with Sertürner's description of morphine's effects in 1817. The isolation of pure, pharmacologically active substances made possible a scientific and quantitative approach to creating and evaluating medicines.[10] In this research tradition, physiological effects were tied to the molecules that triggered them. Doses could be minutely controlled and dose-specific effects monitored. In both academic and industrial settings, chiefly in Germany, chemists learned how to modify molecular structure and produce long series of similar but slightly different molecules. The pharmacologist could then test each in turn for toxicity and therapeutic efficacy. In this painstaking manner, Ehrlich had identified a treatment for syphilis more effective than any yet known, though still associated with undesirable side-effects.

Traditional remedies were reexamined in search of effective molecules for modification and testing. Morphine and codeine were among the earliest alkaloids isolated, and each gave rise to promising semi-synthetics. In this way, new explanatory models were brought to bear on traditional remedies. As the alkaloid was extracted from the complex chemical matrix of plant material, its effects and uses were redefined: not as adjusting system balances of humours and body fluids, but as targeting specific organs or tissues, in response to specific individual diseases and performing, ideally, a single beneficial effect. The aim of drug development was to pare away undesirable effects and isolate desirable ones, aiming at a one-to-one correspondence between a compound and an effect, which could be rendered even more precise through dose titration.

By 1900, a substantial body of literature reflected the accumulated understanding of how chemicals could modify physiological processes. Nevertheless, the methods of drug development were characterized by trial and error, as Ehrlich's exhaustive quest exemplified. New remedies were significant to the extent that they showed comparative advantage over prevailing remedies. However lofty the promise of the magic bullet, the reality was that new drugs came into use because they were somewhat more beneficial than existing ones, or somewhat less toxic.

Practitioners in the first two decades of the twentieth century acknowledged that the scientific revolution in medicine had yielded few new treatment possibilities. Nevertheless, physicians sought to redefine their social relationships with patients by appealing to a scientific basis for authority. With respect to opiates, physicians faced several problems. In the unregulated American market, many preparations containing opium and morphine were freely sold. In 1900, no laws existed to regulate the content or even the labelling and advertising claims for these medicines. The patient choosing to treat his or her own illness or too poor to afford a physician's care faced a welter of exalted claims, some employing the language of science. Were infectious diseases caused by germs? William Radam's Microbe Killer promised to cure all diseases by killing germs. Was radium useful in the treatment of cancer? Rupert Wells' Radol claimed to contain radium and to cure cancer. And myriad preparations claimed to cure narcotic addiction.[11]

Drug development, besides yielding new resources for unscrupulous hawkers, had added to the addiction hazard of opiates. Pure alkaloids and the hypodermic syringe made possible higher effective doses and a quicker path to addiction than was the case with opium taken by mouth. Addiction had become well recognized as a problem connected with opiates, whether self-administered or prescribed by the physician. The profession and the public at large both held the view that physicians' over-prescribing of opiates was the chief cause of addiction.[12]

Against this background, on 7 October 1905, the first of Samuel Hopkins Adams' scathing articles exposing the evils of the patent medicine trade appeared in *Collier's* magazine.[13] These exemplars of the muckraker's art described how unscrupulous charlatans gulled the sick through chicanery, lies, and fraud. Labels made extravagant and false claims that their medicines provided easy cures for the most intractable ills. They lied about the contents of the bottles and powder boxes. Adams described the shady means whereby the purveyors of nostrums assured their access to a gullible public through the press. A common practice was for the advertiser to include in its contract with a newspaper a clause stating that the contract would be cancelled if any law was passed which would render the advertised preparation illegal to sell. Editorial writers were thus put in the position of risking the loss of substantial revenues if they dared to support bills to regulate the sale of drugs.

Adams, like many Progressive reformers, believed that an informed citizenry would be armed to act appropriately in its own interest; his recommendations were to regulate the advertising and labels that deceived the potential purchaser. But he also made a subtle distinction between the individual easily duped and the individual able to make wise decisions when given the facts. He said, 'Intelligent people are not given largely to the use of the glaringly advertised cure-alls, such as Liquozone or Peruna. Nostrums there are, however, which reach the thinking classes as well as the readily gulled.'[14] These were the preparations whose labels failed to disclose the presence of opium. Adams called these the 'most dangerous of all quack medicines, not only in their immediate effect, but because they create enslaving appetites, sometimes obscure and difficult to treat, most often tragically obvious'.[15] Opiates, then, were especially insidious, as they defied even enlightened people's attempts to protect themselves and robbed them of the judgement which was their main tool as effective citizens. Adams assumed that shedding the light of truth on the matter would be sufficient to solve the problem, and Congress substantially agreed when it passed the Pure Food and Drug Act in 1906. The AMA had voiced its support of this legislation in the preceding year.[16] With respect to drugs, this law required that the presence of certain substances, including opiates, be clearly noted on the label. The consumer could then choose knowingly. However, passage of the law did not suffice to solve the problem. Government attempts to prosecute alleged violators met with skilful legal defences, and the struggle to eliminate mislabelled and unsafe medications from the market continued for decades.[17]

For the American physician, the marketing of medicines directly to the public was problematic. Organized medicine was developing a new scientific identity to form the basis not only of knowledge but of social authority and of ethics. This task included many challenges. Allopathic orthodoxy had been staked out, but many irregulars, increasingly considered quacks, had to be eliminated from the field. Self-medication through unregulated sale of medicines must be reduced, both to eliminate the problems connected with misuse and to encourage the public to seek care from physicians rather than to treat themselves. Physicians sought to clarify their channels of service delivery and to determine to what extent they would have a monopoly on dispensing drugs and other treatments. They acted to clean out the pretenders and clean up abuses within the profession. Finally, they created a new rhetoric defining relations between physician and patient. This process meant eliminating traditional remedies that were being discredited by new scientific medicine, and redefining the role of those which had to be retained. The latter group included opiates.

In the early years of the century, leading physicians looked to Progressive ideas as they sought to reform their profession and enhance its prestige. The triumphs of public health workers were prominent in the public mind. For these professionals, the need to change unhealthy behaviours was evident, and public relations and advertising campaigns aimed to improve hygiene in the home and in personal habits. In the period before the First World War, the AMA allied itself with proponents of public health and engaged in spirited campaigns of its own. It reprinted Adams' 'Great American Fraud' articles in book form and distributed thousands of copies. The Council on Pharmacy and Chemistry performed chemical analyses on hundreds of proprietary medicines and published the results in the *Journal of the American Medical Association* (*JAMA*) and in a series of volumes called *Nostrums and Quackery*.[18]

These volumes reveal the rhetorical means whereby physicians sought to undermine certain kinds of claims and establish the authority of others. One aim was to replace an older view of drugs, in which they were to act systemically against a variety of ills, with a newer view in which specific remedies were aimed at the causes of disease. Another was to define the limits of the physician's power given the current state of knowledge, while maintaining the promise that progress would bring greater powers in the future. A third was to relocate authority regarding disease and its cure from the personal experience of patients to the laboratory and the doctor's office. Particular targets included the medicine claiming to 'cure what ails you', from cancer to infectious disease; the medicine which promised to cure diseases for which no cure yet existed, like tuberculosis; the medicine whose ingredients were kept secret; and the patient testimonial.

A standard advertising ploy of the nostrum purveyor was the testimonial in which a grateful customer bore witness to the healing powers of a preparation. The potential new customer was expected to recognize his own ailment in the symptoms outlined in the testimonial and to take hope from the story of relief and cure brought about by the medicine. As early as 1886, the AMA had taken aim at the testimonial as unscientific and irrelevant to the process of cure.[19] In *Nostrums and Quackery*, the most common retort to the testimonial was the 'Laboratory Report', which represented for the AMA publicists the court of final resort. The exalted claims made on behalf of the nostrum were listed; a few testimonials cited; and then the damning evidence of laboratory analysis presented. Medicines were shown to contain chemicals not listed on the label, or to lack ingredients whose presence was claimed. The ingredients present were shown to bear no relation to the disease they purported to cure. The ingredients might be useless, or they might actively worsen the disease. In the case of narcotic addiction, the laboratory evidence was especially appalling: the purported cures actually contained substantial quantities of the addicting drugs themselves.

The effect of pitting the laboratory findings against the personal statements of healing was to replace a vision of disease as a personal and moral crisis with a view of disease as the impersonal result of natural forces. The new bacterial models of disease displaced the individual from the centre of the story. Microbes had a natural life course of their own, and at best the patient was a contender in a two-sided struggle for life.[20] It was also necessary to separate good and true science from bad and spurious science. Claims must be narrowed: no drug could cure every disease, but individual drugs could cure specific, individual diseases by working in a narrowly defined site of action.

Underlying these aims was an ambiguity in the AMA's view of the patient as an informed citizen making choices when faced with illness. In the area of prevention, the citizen's critical role was recognized in the Council on Pharmacy and Chemistry's 1915 report: 'Since it is evident that only by the intelligent cooperation of the laity, can measures necessary for the prevention of disease be successfully introduced, the medical education of the laity was actively promoted by this Association.'[21] However, when illness struck, patients should be knowledgeable enough to recognize the false claims of quacks and nostrum manufacturers, but should also recognize their inability to diagnose, interpret, and treat their own illnesses. The patient should possess the middle-class virtue of being able to spot superstition and humbuggery while trusting to experts to solve the technical problems involved. In short, the patient should be wise enough to know that, when it came to disease, he or she did not know.

The nostrum issue inevitably forced physicians into the commercial world where drugs were bought and sold as commodities. In the pre-war period, a close alliance between pharmaceutical firms and university research laboratories did not yet exist.[22] The AMA sought to clean up the market place and consolidate control over the sale of medications while remaining untainted by commercial gain. In 1884, the Association went on record as opposing the endorsement of medications in advertisements by physicians.[23] One avenue of control was through the advertising policy of the *JAMA*, which might then prove a model for other journals. In 1894, the AMA ruled that *JAMA* should accept no advertising for medications unless a full qualitative and quantitative statement of ingredients was included.[24] In 1906, the Association endorsed acceptance by *JAMA* of advertising for medications approved by the Council on Pharmacy and Chemistry, and it exhorted its members to support other journals with similarly enlightened advertising policies.[25] A stronger resolution in 1915 urged members to withhold support from journals advertising any medications not approved by the Council.[26]

Many of these actions pertained to drugs in general, although, as noted, opiates played a prominent role in the campaign for the 1906 pure food and drug legislation. The main concern with respect to opiates was their potential to cause addiction, and both public and professional attitudes about addiction were undergoing transition in this period. Addicts had typically been portrayed as pitiful individuals who had become enslaved to a vicious habit, often through no fault of their own, although a minority strain contended that addicts possessed some moral or psychological liability which made them prone to become addicted when exposed to opiates. The victims of addiction were more likely to be women than men, they were more likely to be middle aged or old than young, and they tended to come from all parts of the country.[27] The sources of their problem, most observers agreed, was the physician. Drug habits started when physicians prescribed a course of opiates (usually morphine) over several weeks or longer. (Addiction was also a hazard of self-medication, but the labelling requirements of the Pure Food and Drug Act, and continued public education, were making inroads in this area.) The too-free prescribing of opiates not only symbolized old-fashioned, palliative medicine; it had serious iatrogenic consequences. As the medical profession consolidated its claims to be a self-monitoring profession, the reputation for causing addiction must be extirpated. By 1910, American physicians were prescribing opiates less than they had been in earlier decades.[28] Nevertheless, the stigma of association with iatrogenic addiction remained.

The treatment of addiction lay in the same shadowy area as treatment of venereal disease. Patients were often ashamed of the condition, and especially susceptible to the charlatan's promise of quick cure through the anonymous purchase of a nostrum. Many of these preparations contained opiates, as the Council on Pharmacy and Chemistry documented. Although a few state inebriety hospitals existed to treat alcoholics and addicts, more common were private establishments that the AMA viewed with suspicion. Their proprietors traded on the patient's desire for anonymity. They sought referrals from physicians, stressing that addiction was a disease. Like the purveyors of secret nostrums, they were often evasive or silent about the details of the regimen they offered.[29] For respectable physicians, treating addiction as a disease was thus associated with questionable medical practice; yet the availability of even these referral resources may have been welcomed by physicians reluctant to treat addicts themselves.

In 1914, Congress passed the Harrison Narcotic Act. This legislation forbade the sale of opiates and cocaine except as prescribed by a physician and dispensed by a pharmacist. It included requirements that physicians and pharmacists record all prescriptions for opiates and cocaine and forward these to the Treasury Department. The Harrison Act was the first American law to ban the open sale of any drug. The impulse to pass the legislation originated in international concerns: American reformers and diplomats were urging other countries to control the opium trade within their own borders at a time when the US lacked any such controls.[30] For the AMA in the 1910s, limiting imports of opiates to the amounts needed for medical purposes and giving physicians control over who obtained them constituted a desirable policy; the body passed a resolution to this effect in 1912.[31]

The passage of the Harrison Act shifted the emphasis regarding opiates toward intraprofessional concerns. Although the Harrison Act allowed small quantities of some opiates (notably codeine) to be present in medications sold without prescription, generally speaking, the public was protected from indiscriminately swallowing opiates in freely sold nostrums. The task for physicians now consisted of conforming to the new regulations and refining their prescribing practices to avoid censure for prescribing opiates too freely.[32] In 1931, the AMA published *The Indispensable Use of Narcotics*, a volume prepared in collaboration with the National Research Council and containing guidelines for physicians on how to prescribe opiates so as to forestall public criticism.[33] The issue remains alive today.[34]

A pair of Supreme Court decisions in 1919 added an important corollary to the Harrison Act. The Court ruled that to prescribe opiates to an addict in such a manner as to maintain the addiction fell outside the bounds of proper professional practice; such prescribing would therefore constitute a violation of the Harrison Act. Achieving abstinence was declared the only appropriate therapeutic goal in treating addicts. Several cities had established public clinics for the care of the many addicts who were suddenly deprived of legal sources of drugs upon implementation of the Harrison Act, but the Treasury Department closed these in the early 1920s.[35] The Public Health Service, which from the early 1920s undertook extensive research on opiate addiction, opposed any form of ambulatory or clinic treatment of addiction.

The AMA's response to the Harrison Act reveals how problematic the issue of iatrogenic addiction was for physicians and how ready American physicians were to distance themselves from addicts as patients.[36] In the 1920s, physicians were exercising a power previously unparalleled in American history. Rival medical sects such as homeopathy had been virtually eliminated from the field, weakened beyond the power to threaten, or absorbed into the allopathic mould. The foundation of the physician's claim to professionalism was the sacredness of the doctor–patient relationship; the AMA jealously guarded the physician's exclusive right to determine the limits and nature of medical practice. Yet when the Supreme Court presumed to define appropriate and inappropriate treatment for opiate addiction, the AMA did not challenge the decision.

The AMA carefully monitored the enforcement of the Harrison Act as it applied to physicians and objected strongly to certain of its provisions and to some legislative attempts to revise it in the 1920s. For example, the exemption allowing unrestricted sale of medicines containing small amounts of certain opiates was seen as capitulation to the mercenary proprietary drug interests.[37] With respect to treating addicts, however, the AMA substantially agreed with the import of the 1919 Supreme Court decisions. It protested vigorously against convictions of physicians for minor technical violations of the Harrison Act, but it supported the policies of forbidding ambulatory treatment of addicts with resolutions in 1919 and 1924.[38]

In the post-Harrison climate, both the demographics of addiction and attitudes toward addicts were shifting. Beginning even before the passage of the Harrison Act, iatrogenic addiction had begun to decline and a new type of addict was appearing: a young man from the city slums who began taking drugs not because of disease, but in search of thrills.[39] By the time the country was drafting its young men to fight in the European war, this type was well recognized among physicians who worked with addicts, especially in public treatment settings.[40] Opiates and opiate addiction became closely linked with the threat of social disorder through the elaboration of a psychiatric explanation of addiction. The addict became a double-barrelled threat. First, he was a personality type with psychoneurotic deficits who failed to adjust appropriately to expected social roles. Second, once addicted, he lost all moral sense and was essentially beyond the reach of civilized or humane efforts.[41]

This new type of addict posed both a threat and an opportunity for physicians. On the one hand, he was emblematic of the dangers posed by unrestricted sale of opiates. On the other hand, the thrill-seeking addict who purchased drugs on the black market provided a model which did not implicate the physician as a cause of addiction. As concern about this type of addict grew, so did the prevalence of the idea that the addict was not a normal person who became ensnared in the clutches of a terrible substance. Rather, he was a psychiatrically sick individual who was especially susceptible to become addicted when exposed to opiates. Normal persons felt no thrill on taking opiates, but the psychopathic type destined to become an addict felt a special pleasure from them. Addicts could now be described as falling into two classes. 'Accidental' addicts were those normal individuals who became addicted from taking opiates in treatment of illness. They quickly recovered following withdrawal of the drug. 'Vicious' or psychopathic addicts actually sought the drug, and in their case, cure was a dim hope indeed.

The AMA's failure to challenge the federal attempt to define the limits of professional practice suggests that the need to clean medicine's own house of suspect practitioners was felt to be greater than the need to prevent the incursion of lay authority presuming to define some aspect of medical practice. The AMA supported arrest and conviction of physicians who were essentially selling opiate prescriptions for a fee and physicians who were themselves addicted to opiates. From about 1928, a network of communication among the AMA, state medical licensing bodies, and federal narcotics enforcement agents routinely circulated the names of physicians convicted for violating the Harrison Act so that revocation of licensure and publication of the offenders' names in *JAMA* might prevent their resuming their practices.[42] The exoneration of the medical profession from responsibility for the addiction problem was complete by 1940 when a routine AMA response to lay query included the following statement:

We cannot agree with you that the problem of the addict and of addiction is not being properly approached. The major issue in the failure of [the Harrison Act] to meet the situation is due, not to the shortcomings of the medical profession, but rather to the particular nature of the psychological and pathological features of addiction.[43]

OPIATES AS MEDICINE

In 1895, Samuel Potter said in his textbook *Materia Medica, Pharmacy and Therapeutics*, 'Probably no drug in the Materia Medica is so useful as Opium, or has so wide a range of application. At the same time, no drug requires such careful handling, by reason of the many influences which modify its action and uses.' The increasingly problematic nature of opiates as medicine can be traced in materia medica texts and therapeutics manuals published in the US from the 1890s to the 1930s.[44] In these volumes, physicians addressed each other not about the public stature of their profession, but about concrete issues arising during medical practice.

Throughout this period, opiates remained central to the practice of medicine. In the 1890s, opium was said to be 'efficient and convenient in the treatment of all forms of pain'[45] and to have an 'efficiency possessed by no other drug' in the treatment of a long list of painful conditions.[46] In the treatment of the many forms of diarrhoea, opium was 'invaluable', and it was the 'great mainstay' in the treatment of abdominal pain, whether from peritonitis or abdominal surgery.[47] Opiates did not lose their importance as the decades passed. In 1913, opium was 'the most perfect analgesic known'.[48] In 1914, morphine was cited as having 'the power, above all other drugs, to overcome pain and to compel sleep, in spite of everything which ordinarily tends to keep the patient awake'. The writer continued, 'Morphine stands by itself in its power to allay pain, to lessen anxiety and nervous fear, and to change discomfort into comfort.'[49] In the 1920s, morphine remained 'the most efficient of all analgesics' and unrivalled in preventing cough.[50] As late as 1938, a writer stated 'The group of opium alkaloids undoubtedly represents the most important class of all drugs.'[51]

Writers in the 1890s confessed that it would be impossible to list the full range of indications for these indispensable drugs; a partial list might include stomach pain from food or ulcer, peritonitis, meningitis, nausea and vomiting, diarrhoea from many conditions including cholera and dysentery, all forms of inflammation, some mental disorders such as melancholia, cough, asthma, diabetes, emphysema, neuralgia, and a wide range of fevers.[52] A list in the 1920s was only slightly less exhaustive, though, as we shall see, more cautions hedged in the practitioner who would prescribe opiates.[53] Typically, the indications were classed in six broad categories: to relieve pain; to produce sleep; to allay irritation, as in preventing vomiting; to check excessive secretion, as in reducing diarrhoea or bronchial cough; to support the system in low fevers and adynamic states; and as a sudorific.[54]

These all-embracing virtues notwithstanding, opiates presented problems. A writer in 1900 acknowledged that opium 'perhaps best represents the typical symptom medicine, being used almost invariably for the relief of one or more symptoms of disease, rather than for its specific or direct curative action upon the disease itself'.[55] Thus, its ubiquity in therapeutics reflected the limitations of the current state of scientific medicine, which had not yet yielded cures that attacked the causes of diseases. Some slight advances were made in these five decades, though not enough to make wholesale changes in the indications for opiates. For example, in the 1890s, peritonitis was given as an indication without qualification.[56] Within two decades, cautions were urged in the case of peritonitis: the physician should not mask abdominal pain until the need for surgery was determined, and peristalsis should not be slowed or stopped enough to allow the development of intestinal adhesions.[57] Similarly, general recommendations of opiates in cough became more precise: codeine was the opiate of choice, and only irritating, non-productive coughs should be medicated.

The manuals reflect the growing body of pharmacological knowledge. In the earlier manuals, physiological effects were typically grouped according to dose ranges (low, moderate, high).[58] By the 1920s, physiological effects were more likely to be discussed in terms of individual alkaloids. In at least one, effects were linked to what was known about the molecular structure of the component compounds.[59] Nevertheless, this knowledge yielded no revolutionary changes in how opiates were to be used in therapeutics. A manual of 1928 reflects the melange of old and new that characterizes the later manuals. It includes illustrations of the molecular structure of a dozen natural and semi-synthetic opiates and cites scores of animal studies for each known physiological effect. Yet, like traditional materia medica texts, it provides long lists of recipes for individual preparations, including laudanum, liniments, and paregoric. It explains that opiates are most useful when two or more indications are present simultaneously, but its list of indications rivals the earlier contenders in length. It also mentions that calomel and venesection are occasionally called for.[60]

One set of warnings grew steadily more strident: the warning that the practitioner be careful not to induce the opium or morphine habit in the patient. One alert author warned in 1891 against leaving a hypodermic needle in the patient's possession and suggested that morphine relieved pain so profoundly that a habit was always a risk;[61] but far more typically in the early manuals, the danger of inducing a habit was cited as a special danger in connection with a particular indication such as prolonged neuralgia or habitual sleeplessness.[62] In some cases, the habit was even considered an acceptable side-effect. These cases included the old and feeble, and sufferers from diabetes, or from haemorrhages caused by uterine fibroids and cancer.[63] The latter author came to have second thoughts, as in a later edition he warned against prescribing opiates in cases of haemorrhage because of the danger of addiction.[64] By the mid-1920s, warnings about addicting patients were pervasive, and the physician was urged in the case of chronic conditions to resort to opiates only when other remedies had failed. That these authors were also given to statements regarding the unparalleled power of opiates in controlling pain and sleeplessness suggests the problematic status these drugs had attained.[65]

The manuals' discussions of the nature of addiction and how to treat it parallel the rising sentiment in the US that addicts must be sequestered and forbidden to take addictive drugs. Addicts were characterized as liars who had lost all moral sense by most writers who described them.[66] Although some indicated the moral degradation was secondary to the drug use,[67] most did not make this distinction.

The many warnings in the therapeutics discussions about inducing a habit certainly imply that these authors saw physicians' prescribing practices as a significant cause of addiction. More explicit exhortations to the physician to avoid causing iatrogenic addiction were less common but occasionally present.[68] One even warned that a physician should never take an opiate himself unless it was administered by another physician.[69]

Yet opiates remained, in the words of a writer who urged their use only as a last resort, 'the most important class of all drugs'.[70] It was acknowledged in 1900 that however desirable it might be to treat the cause of disease, the use of opiates meant treating symptoms only. Even in the late 1920s and early 1930s, the list of indications remained long and broad. For example, years after the discovery of insulin as a treatment for diabetes, codeine was still recommended for its ability to reduce blood sugar levels.

The trend from the 1890s to the 1930s was a shift in the physician's responsibility in the prescribing of opiates. In the earlier decade, the physician was expected to understand that prescribing opiates carries a risk of causing addiction in certain specific situations. By the 1930s, the physician was exhorted to accept responsibility for preventing addiction through assessment of the patient and extreme care in prescribing. With respect to indications for prescribing opiates, two trends moved in tandem. The growing body of pharmacological knowledge about disease and the dramatically rising concern about addiction both acted to hedge in the indications for opiates.

As regards treatment of opiate addiction, all who discussed it agreed that sudden withdrawal of the drug was potentially dangerous; instead they recommended a course of reduction over seven to twelve days. The addict's lying and manipulative behaviour in attempts to secure drug supplies meant that as a patient, he or she must be closely monitored. Increasingly, this meant treatment in an institution under minute supervision. To manage the addict–patient on any other basis, such as a gradual dose reduction, became untenable. The recommended treatment came to resemble imprisonment. This vision was fully realized with the creation of the Public Health Service Narcotics Hospitals in 1935 and 1938. These institutions were combination prison/hospitals and their inmates included addicted prisoners, probationers, and voluntary inmates. By this time, the weight of medical and scientific authority supported the enforcement policy of removing addicts from American society.

In 1941, the first edition of Louis Goodman and Alfred Gilman's *The Pharmacological Basis of Therapeutics* appeared; it quickly became the standard text of pharmacology in the US. For these writers, morphine was still indispensable for the treatment of pain, and the by-now typical admonitions about avoiding risk of addiction were repeated. In this work, however, the entire discussion of opiates was tightly organized to reflect the laboratory research that had yielded precise dose-response profiles of each morphine effect.[71] Thus, admonitions about avoiding addiction were accompanied by specific recommendations of minimum effective doses for individual indications.

Besides providing the basis for carefully titrated therapeutic doses, dose-response profiles for individual drug effects emphasized the guiding assumption of drug development research: that a drug's actions were a direct function of its molecular structure, and therefore that modifying that structure might yield more useful medications. Research on opiates in the 1930s in the US was dominated by the National Research Council's Committee on Drug Addiction, whose work Goodman and Gilman cited heavily.[72] The committee's chemists had produced hundreds of variations on morphine's molecular structure and its pharmacologists had identified compounds with different combinations of potency for different effects. A specific aim was to identify a compound with morphine's analgesic effects but lacking the addiction potential. Goodman and Gilman cited Metopon, a product of the committee's researches, which was undergoing clinical study. It showed good analgesic potency and a desirable lack of respiratory side-effects. It also proved significantly less addictive than morphine, based on the comparatively mild symptoms which followed withdrawal after continuous administration. Addiction had become, for the pharmacologist, a measurable side-effect like any other.

ACKNOWLEDGEMENTS

The research for this essay was supported by a travel grant from the Graduate Division, University of California, San Francisco. I am grateful to Christopher Lawrence for his comments on an earlier draft of this essay.

NOTES

1 On the rise of medicine and public health as paradigmatic of the emergence of the new professional middle class in the US, see Robert H. Wiebe, *The Search for Order: 1877–1920* (New York, 1967).

2 On the transformation of medical education in the US, see Kenneth M. Ludmerer, *Learning to Heal: The Development of American Medical Education* (New York, 1985), and William G. Rothstein, *American Medical Schools and the Practice of Medicine* (New York, 1987).

3 See Morris Vogel, *Invention of the Modern Hospital* (Chicago, 1980), on early initiatives to reform Harvard Medical School along the lines of the German model.

4 On the political activities of the American Medical Association, see James G. Burrow, *A.M.A.: Voice of American Medicine* (Baltimore, 1963).

5 On the development of laboratory methods in the German pharmaceutical industry, see Georg Meyer-Thurow, 'The Industrialization of Invention: A Case Study from the German Chemical Industry', *Isis*, 73 (1982), pp. 363–81.

6 AMA, *1846–1958 Digest of Official Actions* (Chicago: AMA, 1958), p. 183.

7 W. T. Councilman, W. W. Grant and M. L. Harris, 'Special Report on the Council on Pharmacy and Chemistry', *American Medical Association Bulletin*, 10 (15 May 1915), p. 338.

8 *Ibid.*, p. 331.

9 *Ibid.*, p. 335n.

10 John Parascandola, 'Reflections on the History of Pharmacology', *Pharmacy in History*, 22 (1980), pp. 131–40.

11 On the sale of nostrums and patent medicines in this period, see James Harvey Young, *The Medical Messiahs: A Social History of Health Quackery in Twentieth-Century America* (Princeton, 1967).

12 On the prominence of the view that physicians were largely responsible for addiction, see Charles E. Terry and Mildred Pellens, *The Opium Problem* (New York: Bureau of Social Hygiene, 1928), ch. 3. Terry and Pellens, in a project funded by the Rockefeller-supported Bureau of Social Hygiene, surveyed the writings of physicians and scientists on both sides of the Atlantic on addiction, from the 1870s through the 1920s. Their work remains an important authoritative source on scientific views of this phenomenon. See also David Musto, *The American Disease: Origins of Narcotic Control* (New Haven, 1973), pp. 93–8. Musto is equally indispensable on the passage of legislation regulating the sale of opiates.

13 The series contained five articles under the general title, 'The Great American Fraud': 'Part I', *Collier's* (7 Oct. 1905), pp. 14–15, 29; 'Part II: Peruna and the Bracers', *Collier's* (28 Oct. 1905), pp. 17–19; 'Part III: Liquozone', *Collier's* (18 Nov. 1905), pp. 20–1; 'Part IV: The Subtle Poisons', *Collier's* (2 Dec. 1905), pp. 16–18; 'Part V: Preying on the Incurables', *Collier's* (13 Jan. 1906), pp. 18–20.

14 Adams, 'Subtle Poisons', p. 16.

15 *Ibid.*

16 AMA, *Digest of Official Actions*, p. 183.

17 Young, *The Medical Messiahs*.

18 AMA, *Nostrums and Quackery*, vol. I, 2nd edn (Chicago: AMA Press, 1912); Arthur J. Cramp, ed., *Nostrums and Quackery*, vol. II (Chicago: AMA Press, 1921).

19 AMA, *Digest of Official Actions*, p. 181.

20 See, for example, Barbara Gutmann Rosenkrantz, *Public Health and the State: Changing Views in Massachusetts, 1852–1936* (Cambridge, Mass., 1972), p. 116.

21 Councilman *et al.*, 'Special Report', p. 331.

22 John P. Swann, *Academic Scientists and the Pharmaceutical Industry* (Baltimore, 1988).

23 AMA, *Digest of Official Actions*, pp. 180–1.

24 *Ibid.*, p. 182.

25 *Ibid.*, p. 184.

26 *Ibid.*, p. 187.

27 On the shifting demographics of opiate addiction in the period covered by this paper, see David T. Courtwright, *Dark Paradise: Opiate Addiction in America before 1940* (Cambridge, Mass., 1982).

28 *Ibid.*, p. 54.

29 Examples of correspondence and promotional literature describing medications and establishments for the treatment of addiction can be found in the AMA Historical Health Fraud and Alternative Medicine Collection, AMA Archives, Chicago, Ill., Box 0823 Folder 04; Box 0517 Folder 09. Cited hereafter as AMA Health Fraud Collection.

30 Musto, *The American Disease*.

31 AMA, *Digest of Official Actions*, p. 501.

32 For an example of the efforts of state medical society to translate the requirements of the law into specific guidelines for physicians, see Cornelius F. Collins, 'The Law and the Narcotic Addict', *Long Island Medical Journal*, 13 (1919), pp. 272–9; Royal S. Copeland, 'The Attitude of the Health Department', *Long Island Medical Journal*, 13 (1919), pp. 269–72; Sara Graham-Mulhall, 'The New York State Narcotic Commission', *Long Island Medical Journal*, 13 (1919), pp. 279–84; Benjamin A. Mathews, 'Medical Practice as Affected by the Harrison Law', *Long Island Medical Journal*, 13 (1919), pp. 284–95.

33 Various authors, *The Indispensable Use of Narcotics* (Chicago: AMA 1931).

34 See, for example, the *Journal of Psychoactive Drugs*, 23 (October–November 1991), p. 4.

35 Musto, *The American Disease*.

36 See also *ibid.*, pp. 82–5.

37 Arthur J. Cramp (Director of the AMA's Bureau of Investigation) to J. Marks, 10 May 1918; Cramp to Benjamin Perry, 27 August 1918. Both in AMA Health Fraud Collection, Box 0302 Folder 03.

38 AMA, *Digest of Official Actions*, pp. 502–3.

39 Courtwright, *Dark Paradise*.

40 The type was well described in the diagnostic categories for psychiatrists screening First World War recruits and draftees. See Pearce Bailey, Frankwood E. Williams, and Paul O. Komora, 'In the United States', in *Neuropsychiatry*, vol. x of *The Medical Department of the United States Army in the World War* (Washington: US Surgeon General's Office, 1929).

41 This view contended with physiological explanations of addiction and with more humane views of the addict until the 1920s. It was consolidated as the official enforcement view and dominant scientific model through the work of Lawrence Kolb, a Public Health Service psychiatrist. Kolb's views were offered in a series of articles appearing in 1925: 'Pleasure and Deterioration from Narcotic Addiction', *Mental Hygiene*, 9 (1925), pp. 699–724; 'Relation of Intelligence to Etiology of Drug Addiction', *American Journal of Psychiatry*, 5 (1925),

pp. 163–7; 'Types and Characteristics of Drug Addicts', *Mental Hygiene*, 9 (1925), pp. 300–13.

42 Holman Taylor to William C. Woodward, 21 January 1928, AMA Health Fraud Collection, Box 0321 Folder 09. The Collection contains several boxes of such correspondence from the late 1920s through the early 1960s.

43 AMA to Catharine H. Griggs, 8 January 1940, AMA Health Fraud Collection, Box 0321 Folder 12.

44 The following works were reviewed (they are listed in chronological order of the first edition cited for each author): Roberts Bartholow, *A Practical Treatise on Materia Medica and Therapeutics*, 7th edn (New York, 1890); idem, *A Practical Treatise on Materia Medica and Therapeutics*, 12th edn (New York, 1906); H. C. Wood, *Therapeutics: Principles and Practice*, 7th edn (Philadelphia, 1890); Horatio C. Wood and Horatio C. Wood, Jr, *Therapeutics: Its Principles and Practice*, 13th edn (Philadelphia, 1906); John V. Shoemaker, *Materia Medica and Therapeutics*, vol. II of *A Treatise of Materia Medica, Pharmacology, and Therapeutics* (Philadelphia, 1891); idem, *A Practical Treatise on Materia Medica and Therapeutics*, 6th edn (Philadelphia, 1906); Samuel O. L. Potter, *Handbook of Materia Medica, Pharmacy, and Therapeutics*, 5th edn (Philadelphia, 1895); idem, *Therapeutics, Materia Medica, and Pharmacy*, 11th edn (Philadelphia, 1909); idem, *Therapeutics Materia Medica and Pharmacy*, 13th edn (Philadelphia, 1917); W. Hale White, *Materia Medica: Pharmacy, Pharmacology and Therapeutics*, 4th American edn (Philadelphia, 1899); George Frank Butler, *A Textbook of Materia Medica, Therapeutics and Pharmacology*, 3rd edn (Philadelphia, 1900); idem, *A Text-Book of Materia Medica Pharmacology and Therapeutics*, 6th edn (Philadelphia, 1908); William Schlief, *Materia Medica, Therapeutics Pharmacology and Pharmacognosy*, 3rd edn (Philadelphia, 1907); Reynold Webb Wilcox, *Materia Medica and Therapeutics*, 8th edn (Philadelphia, 1913); idem, *Materia Medica and Therapeutics*, 12th edn (Philadelphia, 1929); Walter A. Bastedo, *Materia Medica: Pharmacology: Therapeutics, Prescription Writing*, 1st edn (Philadelphia, 1914); idem, *Materia Medica, Pharmacology, Therapeutics and Prescription Writing*, 3rd edn (Philadelphia, 1932); A. A. Stevens, *A Text-Book of Therapeutics*, 6th edn (Philadelphia, 1923); Alfred Martinet, *Clinical Therapeutics*, vols. I and II (Philadelphia, 1925); Francis W. Palfrey, *The Art of Medical Treatment* (Philadelphia, 1925); Solomon Solis-Cohen and Thomas Stotesbury Githens, *Pharmacotherapeutics, Materia Medica and Drug Action* (New York, 1928); Eldin V. Lynn, *Pharmaceutical Therapeutics*, 1st edn (New York, 1929); idem, *Pharmaceutical Therapeutics*, 2nd edn (New York, 1938). As this list represents a sampling rather than an exhaustive catalogue of available texts, the conclusions drawn are about general trends. No claim is made to identify the first appearance in the literature of any given point.

45 Shoemaker, *Materia Medica*, p. 786.

46 Potter, *Handbook*, 5th edn, p. 317.

47 White, *Materia Medica*, 4th edn, p. 336.

48 Wilcox, *Materia Medica*, 8th edn, p. 734.

49 Bastedo, *Materia Medica*, 1st edn, p. 357.

50 *Ibid.*

51 Lynn, *Pharmaceutical Therapeutics*, 2nd edn, p. 274.

52 Bartholow, *Practical Treatise*, 7th edn, pp. 581–9.

53 Solis-Cohen and Githens, *Pharmacotherapeutics*, pp. 1684–95.

54 This system appears in Wood, *Therapeutics*, 7th edn, pp. 164–6, and Butler, *Textbook*, 3rd edn, p. 453. Variants appear as late as 1928 in Solis-Cohen and Githens, *Pharmacotherapeutics*, pp. 1685–6.

55 Butler, *Textbook*, 3rd edn, p. 453.

56 'In *peritonitis*, whether *puerperal, traumatic*, or the extension of *intestinal inflammation*, no fact of therapeutics is better established than the curative power of opium.' Bartholow, *Practical Treatise*, 7th edn, p. 584.

57 Wilcox, *Materia Medica*, 8th edn, p. 738; Solis-Cohen and Githens, *Pharmacotherapeutics*, pp. 1689–90.

58 For example, Bartholow, *Practical Treatise*, 7th edn, p. 576.

59 For example, 'While morphine, codeine and thebaine have a stimulant action on the intestinal motions . . . the other opium alkaloids which have a benzyl-isoquinoline nucleus, have just the opposite effect', Solis-Cohen and Githens, *Pharmacotherapeutics*, p. 1674.

60 Solis-Cohen and Githens, *Pharmacotherapeutics*.

61 Shoemaker, *Materia Medica*, p. 786.

62 Bartholow, *Practical Treatise*, 7th edn, p. 588; Wood, *Therapeutics*, 7th edn, p. 164.

63 Wood, *Therapeutics*, 7th edn, pp. 165–6; Potter, *Handbook*, 5th edn, pp. 317–18.

64 Potter, *Therapeutics*, 13th edn.

65 The first such sweeping warning in the manuals surveyed appears in Wilcox, *Materia Medica*, 8th edn, p. 740. Wilcox accompanied his warning with the statement that indications for opiates were too numerous to list completely. Solis-Cohen and Githens, *Pharmacotherapeutics*, p. 1694, also couples a blanket warning regarding chronic pain or insomnia with statements that no other medications can alleviate these conditions as well as opiates.

66 Wood, *Therapeutics*, 7th edn, p. 169; White, *Materia Medica*, p. 340; Wilcox, *Materia Medica*, 8th edn, p. 745; Bastedo, *Materia Medica*, p. 364; Solis-Cohen and Githens, *Pharmacotherapeutics*, pp. 263, 1671. The latter authors cite a physician addict who stated that 'We are all liars'.

67 Butler, *Textbook*, 3rd edn, p. 451.

68 *Ibid.*; Stevens, *Text-Book*, p. 91.

69 Palfrey, *Art of Medical Treatment*, p. 130.

70 Lynn, *Pharmaceutical Therapeutics*, 1st edn, p. 283.

71 Louis Goodman and Alfred Gilman, *The Pharmacological Basis of Therapeutics* (New York, 1941), pp. 186–223.

72 The work of the National Research Council's Committee on Drug Addiction in the 1930s is discussed in Caroline Jean Acker, 'Social Problems and Scientific Opportunities: The Case of Opiate Addiction in the United States, 1920–1940' (PhD diss., University of California, San Francisco, 1993).

SEVEN

CHANGES IN ALCOHOL USE AMONG NAVAJOS AND OTHER INDIANS OF THE AMERICAN SOUTHWEST

STEPHEN J. KUNITZ AND JERROLD E. LEVY

INTRODUCTION

FROM the time of earliest contact, it has been observed that the beverage alcohol introduced by Europeans had devastating consequences on Native North Americans. High rates of devastation have persisted into the present, as Figure 1 indicates. The data displayed there show that the age-adjusted rate of alcohol-related deaths[1] had declined among Indians since the late 1960s, but increased in the late 1980s and is 5.4 times higher than it is for all races in the United States. The category of alcohol-related deaths does not include accidents, which was the second leading cause of death among Indians and Alaska Natives in 1988 and occurred at slightly more than twice the frequency as among all races in the United States. Slightly more than 50% of accidental deaths of Indians involve motor vehicles, and at least half of these are estimated to be due to alcohol abuse. Clearly, although the long-term trend of deaths involving alcohol seems to be a convergence between Indians and non-Indians, the differences are still substantial.

There have been a variety of explanations for the high rates of alcohol-related problems among Indians, none of which necessarily excludes any of the others.[2] Perhaps the oldest in one form or another is that Indians cannot hold their liquor because biologically they are unable to do so. This explanation continues to be the subject of empirical scientific investigation, and is based upon the assumption that there is some genetic mechanism that is a necessary cause of alcohol abuse: without such a mechanism Indians would not have the problems with alcohol that they do. A recent review indicates, however, that no compelling evidence for the hypothesis has yet been found.[3]

A second explanation of the high rates of alcohol abuse among Indians is that acculturation, stress, and poverty are the causes.[4] According to this explanation, Indians drink excessively because their

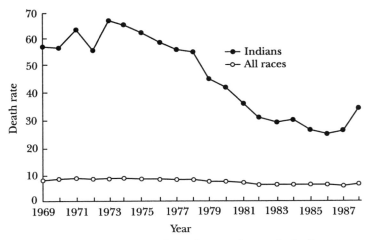

Figure 1   Age-adjusted death rates due to alcoholism
Source: Indian Health Service, *Trends in Indian Health 1991* (Washington, DC: US Department of Health and Human Services, Public Health Service, 1991).

own societies and cultures are no longer intact, and they are deprived of access to the valued goods of the society which has engulfed them.

A third and yet more recent explanation has been that the way people behave when they have consumed alcohol is learned. In the context within which Indians learned to use alcohol – a frontier situation in which social restraints were loosened and alcohol use was regarded as time out from one's normal obligations – the flamboyant, unrestrained, and sometimes violent behaviour that is usually thought to characterize Indian drinking was, and continues to be, the norm.[5]

We have been impressed with how diverse Indian populations are in respect of social organization, culture, ecological adaptation, and history of contact with Europeans, a diversity that we think is reflected in the heterogeneity of alcohol uses and its sequelae. We have argued elsewhere, for example, that what was learned about drunken behaviour was not simply a product of watching the effect of alcohol upon Euro-American frontiersmen, but was mediated by the culture of particular Indian groups, as well as by ease of access to alcohol.[6] Thus, while the rates of alcohol-related deaths are on average high for Indians compared with non-Indians, the great differences among equally poor Indian populations suggest that something more than simply a biological defect or poverty is likely to be at work. Several writers, ourselves included, have argued that social organization is an extremely important explanatory variable, and that tightly integrated sedentary agricultural peoples are likely to be less flamboyant in their use of alcohol than more loosely integrated hunter-gatherers, to be less individualistic and more constrained by community social controls, and to be less likely to act out impulsively.[7]

In this essay we should like to accomplish several tasks. First, we shall illustrate some of the heterogeneity of alcohol use and its consequences that is observed among regional groupings of Indian tribes, among tribes within one region of the country, and within one tribe. Second, we shall describe some of the temporal changes in alcohol use and its sequelae within the Navajo population. And third, we shall describe patterns of alcohol use and its consequences over the life course among several groups of Navajo Indians followed for more than two decades. Our purpose is to suggest what some of the socio-cultural determinants of heterogeneity and secular change have been and some of the questions they raise for the future in respect of prevention, treatment, and research.

THE SEQUELAE OF ALCOHOL USE AMONG INDIAN POPULATIONS

Health care for many Indians in the United States is provided free of charge by the Indian Health Service of the US Public Health Service. For administrative purposes, the populations receiving health services are divided into twelve regions, all but one of which are west of the Mississippi River. Table 1 displays selected socio-economic and mortality data from each of the regions.[8] It is clear that there is a substantial range in median family income, educational levels, and rates of death from accidental and alcohol-related causes. Not surprisingly, there is a strong positive correlation (Spearman's $r = 0.601$, $p < 0.05$) between the two death rates. There is also a strong negative correlation ($r = -0.63$, $p < 0.05$) between the accident rate and levels of education. There is a less strong positive correlation ($r = 0.513$, $p < 0.05$) between income and education and even weaker correlations between income and accidental ($r = -0.441$, $p > 0.05$) and alcohol-related ($r = -0.42$, $p > 0.05$) deaths. There is no relationship whatever between education and alcohol-related deaths. Thus, while the associations are generally in the expected directions – where income is low, death rates tend to be high – the correlations are not particularly strong.

Of course, populations as large as those in these administrative regions are for the most part far from homogeneous. We thus consider death rates from various alcohol-related conditions in various service

Table 1. *Education, income, and mortality rates, Native Americans and Alaska Natives, 1986–88, by area*

| Area | Median household income | Median years of education, > 25 years of age | Age adjusted death rates/ 100,000 pop. | |
			Accidents	Alcoholism
Navajo	$8,412	9.3	160.7	36.6
Tucson	$9,432	11.0	219.9	66.6
Aberdeen	$9,625	11.9	129.0	69.9
Bemidji	$10,464	11.9	99.2	32.8
Billings	$10,967	12.2	139.4	57.8
Nashville	$11,471	11.8	72.4	24.3
Oklahoma	$11,579	12.2	44.8	9.5
Albuquerque	$12,226	12.2	120.2	56.4
Phoenix	$12,295	12.3	128.8	64.5
California	$13.235	12.4	50.6	15.2
Portland	$13,563	12.4	91.6	39.5
Alaska	$15,750	9.3	153.3	22.5

Source: Indian Health Service, *Trends in Indian Health 1991* (Washington, DC: US Department of Health and Human Services, Public Health Service, 1991).

units, which are administrative units within the larger regions we have just discussed. The service units we have selected are all in the Southwest and are relatively homogeneous in respect of tribal composition. Table 2 displays death rates from accidents and cirrhosis of the liver from 1975 to 1977.[9] Notice that there is great variability in death rates among tribes; more than three-fold for accidents, more than ten-fold for cirrhosis of the liver. Some order is evident, however. Apaches tend to have substantially higher accident death rates than Pueblos (Hopis and Eastern Pueblos). This is in accordance with what we have suggested above, that loosely organized tribes like the Apaches will have more flamboyant alcohol-related drinking behaviour than the tightly organized, relatively highly controlled sedentary agriculturalists like the Pueblos. The Navajos, an Apachean group which has been heavily influenced by Pueblo contacts, seem to be intermediate between the Pueblo and Apache groups. The River Yumans are an agricultural people loosely organized into tribes which, however, had 'a minimum of organization for social control'.[10]

No discernible pattern is evident for cirrhosis, a topic to which we shall return below. It does appear that the low rates among the Navajos and Hopis may be the result in part of relatively limited access to alcoholic beverages, since their reservations tend to be more remote from sources of supply than the others. Indeed, several other equally

Table 2. *Death rates per 100,000 from accidents and cirrhosis of the liver, IHS service units, 1975–7*

Service unit	Tribe	Accidents	Cirrhosis
Mescalero	Apache	317.8	229.5
Keams Canyon	Hopi, some Navajo	102.1	18.6
San Carlos	Apache	212.2	57.9
Whiteriver	Apache	196.0	58.8
Santa Fe	Eastern Pueblo, some Apache	91.6	48.2
Colorado River	Yuman	124.3	55.2
Navajo Area (inc. 8 service units)	Navajos	186.3	21.6

Source: Indian Health Service, *Selected Vital Statistics for Indian Health Service Areas and Service Units, 1972 to 1977*, DHEW Publication No. (HSA) 79-1005 (Rockville, Md.: US Department of Health, Education, and Welfare, Public Health Service, 1979).

remote tribes (the San Carlos and Whiteriver Apaches) have legalized the sale of liquor, which assures that it is readily available.

A second example comes from a study of the consequences of alcohol use among a number of Indian tribes in Oklahoma. Tribes in eastern Oklahoma had substantially lower rates of alcohol-related arrests and deaths than did Indians in western Oklahoma. The Indians in the East had originally been farmers and woodsmen (Creek, Cherokee, Seminole, Chickasaw, and Choctaw) whereas the tribes in the West had been hunters on the Plains (Cheyenne, Arapaho, Kiowa, Apache, Comanche among others).[11] These data indicate, as do those above, that traditional patterns of social organization and culture may have continuing relevance for understanding patterns of alcohol use and the epidemiology of its various sequelae. In addition, however, it was observed that high rates of arrest for public intoxication as well as alcohol-related deaths are related to high areas of unemployment.

A third example comes from a study of the epidemiology of Fetal Alcohol Syndrome and Fetal Alcohol Effect. These are recently described conditions that result from the ingestion of alcohol during pregnancy. A variety of physical and cognitive deficits have been described in affected children. May and his colleagues have shown that the incidence rates of Fetal Alcohol Syndrome and Fetal Alcohol Effect differ among tribes: Navajos and Puebloes have lower rates (3.6 per 1,000 and 4.4 per 1,000 respectively) than do Eastern Apaches and Southern Utes, both of which were band level hunting groups (27.7 per 1,000).[12] Thus alcohol use among women of childbearing age seems to vary with social organization in the same way as do other sequelae of alcohol use.

Finally, our own work among Navajo and Hopi Indians suggests that there are important differences between these two peoples in drinking behaviour and in the consequences of drinking. We have already observed that in the early 1970s reported death rates from cirrhosis of the liver were about the same. The problem with these data is that many of the Hopis who died of cirrhosis had moved off their reservation to border towns which were within the Navajo Area. Since tribal affiliation is generally not listed on the death certificate, and not tabulated when it is, the only designation available is race: Indian, Caucasian, Black, and so on. Thus, an Indian dying in the Navajo Area is assumed to be a Navajo. In most instances this is a reasonable assumption. In the present instance, however, it is not.

By searching Indian Health Service hospital records, which do record tribal membership, and by interviewing survivors of people who had died, we found an average annual death rate from cirrhosis for Hopis in 1965–7 of 43.3 per 100,000. The Navajo rate at the same time was about 14 per 100,000. In the 1970s the Hopi rate declined to about 37.3 and the Navajo rate increased to about 21 per 100,000.[13] We have suggested that among Hopis drinking is regarded as a highly deviant act. It is pursued privately and, if it cannot be contained by the usual mechanisms of social control, the deviant drinker is likely to be expelled from the community. Thus the cirrhotics who died while living off reservation tended to be from villages in which traditional mechanisms of social control were still functioning. The result was diminished support from family and friends, and we believe the assumption by the drinker of a self-image as someone beyond the pale and not redeemable.

Among Navajos, on the other hand, drinking has not been regarded as deviant in the same fashion. We shall discuss Navajo patterns below and will simply say here that highly visible group drinking has been common and in the past has not been considered a problem calling for the exercise of strict mechanisms of social control. Thus many Navajos, particularly men, drink a great deal, often become intoxicated and have accidents as a result, but for the most part they do not become social isolates. The result seems to be that their heavy drinking does not as commonly progress to alcoholic cirrhosis.

Thus far we have shown that when considering American Indians as a population, we observe both temporal changes in the sequelae of alcohol use as well as internal differentiation. Both sets of observations suggest that alcohol use is not a single phenomenon but rather is heterogeneous and responsive to a variety of forces, among which culture and social organization continue to be important. We shall also observe heterogeneity as we narrow our focus to a single tribe, the

Table 3. *Mortality rates per 100,000 due to various causes, Navajo Indians, 1960s–1980s*

Cause	1960s	1970s	1980s
Alcoholic cirrhosis	(a) 6.2–7.1[a] (b) 14.1 (c) 15.1–17.3	18.1–20.6[b]	9.7–11.0[c]
Motor vehicle accidents	(a) 54.6–62.8[d] (b) 66.0–75.5	114.8–130.6[e]	77.3–88.0[f]

[a] (a) S. J. Kunitz, J. E. Levy, and M. Everett, 'Alcoholic Cirrhosis among the Navajo', *Quarterly Journal of Studies on Alcohol*, 30 (1969), pp. 672–85: years 1965–7. (b) IHS, *Indian Health Trends and Services. 1970 Edition* (Rockville, Md.: PHS Publication No. 2092, Office of Program Planning and Evaluation, Program Analysis and Statistics Branch, Indian Health Service, US Department of Health, Education and Welfare, 1971): years 1965–7. (c) IHS, *1968 Indian Vital Statistics: Navajo Area* (Tucson, Ariz.: Health Program Systems Center, Indian Health Service, US Dept HEW, 1970): year 1968.
[b] S. J. Kunitz, *Disease Change and the Role of Medicine: The Navajo Experience* (Berkeley, Calif., 1983), p. 104: average annual rates, 1972–8.
[c] Navajo Area Indian Health Service, unpublished data provided by Dr Michael Everett, average annual rate 1985–8. These figures are for alcoholic liver disease (ICDA 9 codes 571.0–571.3). If codes 571.5 (cirrhosis without mention of alcohol) and 571.6 (biliary cirrhosis) are included, the rate increases to 11.9–13.6.
[d] (a) R. C. Brown *et al.*, 'The Epidemiology of Accidents among the Navajo Indians', *Public Health Reports*, 85 (1970), pp. 881–8: for single year 1968. (b) IHS 1970, for 1968, see n. 1 above.
[e] Kunitz, see n. 2 above, pp. 101–2. Average annual rate 1972–8, recalculated using IHS population figures, from Navajo Area Indian Health Service, *1986 Natality–Mortality Report* (Window Rock, Ariz.: Office of Program Planning and Development, NAIHS, US Public Health Services, 1989).
[f] Navajo Area Indian Health Service, unpublished data, average annual rates 1985–8.

Navajo, and once again consider both secular trends and internal differentiation of patterns and sequelae of alcohol use.

THE NAVAJO

The changing epidemiology of cirrhosis and motor vehicle accidents

In Table 3 we provide estimates of the Navajo death rate from cirrhosis in the 1960s, 1970s, and 1980s.[14] Significantly, no matter what source of data one uses, death rates from cirrhosis increased from the 1960s to the 1970s and declined just as significantly from the 1970s to the 1980s.

Age-specific rates in the 1970s showed a pattern for both males and females that was very different from the one observed among Anglo-Americans. Navajo deaths peaked in the 30s whereas Anglo deaths peaked in the 50s. The age groups that accounted for the great elevation

Table 4. *Average annual Navajo death rates per 100,000 from alcoholic cirrhosis, 1972–8 and 1985–8, by age and sex*

Age group	Males		Females	
	1972–8[a]	1985–8[b]	1972–8[a]	1985–8[b]
25–34	62	49.7	28	27.9
35–44	103	50.2	58	20.7
45–54	46	55.0	47	35.0
55–64	52	0.0	31	33.3
> 65	23	13.2	33	0.0

[a] Kunitz, *Disease Change and the Role of Medicine*, p. 104. These rates are based upon what we believe to be high population estimates. The rates might therefore be as much as 15% higher.
[b] Calculated from unpublished data from the Navajo Area Indian Health Service. The population estimates are likely to be low. Higher population estimates would produce rates as much as 15% lower. Cirrhosis includes alcoholic fatty liver, alcoholic hepatitis, alcoholic cirrhosis, and alcoholic liver damage, but excludes non-alcoholic cirrhosis (11 male and 6 female deaths, the youngest of whom died in their early 40s, the majority in their 50s and 60s).

in the 1970s were men 25–44 and women 25–54.[15] These patterns changed in the late 1980s, as Table 4 indicates. Considering the uncertainty of the population estimates and the small size of the oldest age groups, great confidence cannot be placed in the precise rates we have reported. What we do think is substantively important, however, is the very large drop in the rates for both women and men in the age group 35–44. In our previous work we have been impressed that the very high age-specific rates of violent and alcohol-related deaths declined in the early 40s as if men in particular had passed a crisis point and entered a new phase of their lives.[16] We were writing of people born in the 1930s and earlier. The people 34–44 in 1985–8 were born between the late 1930s and early 1950s; it is not clear what in the historical experience of this cohort may have caused a change of such magnitude.

In general, the evidence suggests that by the 1980s mortality from cirrhosis had declined precipitously and roughly paralleled national trends.[17] Moreover, it was especially dramatic among men. We had estimated the average annual rates for men and women in 1972–8 as 21.8 and 14.7 respectively, based upon high population estimates.[18] The comparable figures in 1985–8 are 11.0 and 8.5, a decrease of 50% among men and 42% among women.[19]

When we consider accidents, the leading cause of death among Navajos, we observe similar patterns. Motor vehicle accidents comprise

Table 5. *Average annual Navajo motor vehicle accidents death rates per 100,000 by age and sex, 1972–8 and 1985–8*

	Males		Females	
Age group	1972–8[a]	1985–8[b]	1972–8[a]	1985–8[b]
< 10	32–7	26–30	29–33	15–18
10–14	27–32	16–19	11–13	4–5
15–24	287–330	198–233	78–90	43–50
25–34	392–450	286–337	93–107	73–86
35–44	225–59	213–51	88–101	53–62
45–54	202–32	85–100	72–83	36–42
55–64	249–86	125–47	31–6	43–50
> 65	201–31	129–52	53–61	70–82

[a] Kunitz, *Disease Change and the Role of Medicine*, p. 102.
[b] Based upon unpublished data from the Navajo Area Indian Health Service.

the single largest proportion of accidental deaths, and it is said that many if not most of them are alcohol related. Table 3 displays estimates of average annual rates during the 1960s from two different sources. They range from 54 to 75 per 100,000 and stand in stark contrast to the following decade, when the average annual number of motor vehicle accident deaths was 151 (from 1972 through 1978), and the average annual rate was between 114.8 and 130.6 per 100,000. As in the case of cirrhosis, this appears to represent a real increase and is not simply a result of deficient case ascertainment in the 1960s. The rates were three times higher for men than women, they were highest for men in the 25–34 age group, but in fact they were remarkably high starting in the late teens and going right through to the 60s. Multiple regression analyses of both the average annual motor vehicle accident mortality rates and hospitalization rates due to motor vehicle accidents suggested that they were highest in the most densely settled areas of the Reservation.[20]

Again as in the case of cirrhosis, there was a dramatic decline of about one third in deaths from this cause from the 1970s to the 1980s. The sex ratio remained unchanged, however. About three times as many men as women died in motor vehicle accidents (men, 119.6–136.2; women, 36.7–41.8 per 100,000 average annual rate 1985–8). This pattern of decreasing rates of death since the 1970s parallels the national pattern, just as cirrhosis deaths do.[21]

Unlike cirrhosis deaths, however, which showed a particularly dramatic decline in the 35–44 age group, there was a general decline of motor vehicle accident deaths in virtually all age categories (see

Table 5). This is not surprising considering that not all fatal accidents are alcohol related (see below), and that when an accident does occur, people of all ages and degree of sobriety may be involved, whether the driver(s) was drunk or not. The assumption underlying discussions of motor vehicle accidents is that they are caused primarily by drunken drivers. Only one study has attempted a careful analysis of the association, however. Katz and May analysed police reports of motor vehicle accidents on the Navajo Reservation for the years 1973–5.[22] Even these data are subject to potential downward bias because blood alcohol levels were not known. Instead the investigating officer checked a box stating that the subject had been drinking, or left it blank if the subject had not been drinking. Katz and May concluded that, 'For Indian cases the proportion of alcohol involvement for single-vehicle, multiple-vehicle, and single-vehicle/pedestrian accidents is 41 percent, 46 percent, and 44 percent respectively.'[23] They went on to point out that studies in other populations had reported higher rates of alcohol involvement in fatal motor vehicle accidents but that those studies had used blood alcohol levels, not simply the investigating officers' impressions, which may well have missed subtle signs of intoxication. Nonetheless, if even half the accidents are associated with drunken driving, the carnage due to alcohol use is substantial because the total rate is so high.[24] On the other hand, it should be clear that many other forces are at work to produce high accident rates, including poorly engineered roads, poorly maintained vehicles, inadequate driver training, and the great distances many people must drive for work, shopping, and medical care, not to mention for alcohol. Thus to invoke alcohol abuse as the major determinant not only oversimplifies the problem but has the effect of blaming the victim for what may often be environmental conditions beyond his or her control.

It is unfortunate that as yet there has been no repeat of the study by Katz and May. In light of the decline in alcoholic cirrhosis and the parallel decline in motor vehicle fatalities, it would be important to know if changes in alcohol consumption patterns are responsible for the reduction in accidents as they must be for alcoholic cirrhosis.

The changing prevalence of alcohol use

In a field study from the mid-1960s[25] we reported the drinking status of people in three groups: the adult members of an extended kin group in a rural area, called the Plateau Group; a random sample of adults living in the Reservation administrative and wage work centre of Tuba City, Arizona, called the South Tuba sample; and all the Navajo

Table 6. *The prevalence of alcohol use in several samples of Navajo men and women, 1960s and 1980s*

Drinking status	Plateau (1966)[a]	South Tuba (1966)[a]	Flagstaff (1967)[a]	Winslow (1984)[b]
Women				
Life-long abstainer	9 (37.5%)	9 (64.3%)	20 (66.7%)	
Stopped drinking	14 (58.3%)	4 (28.6%)	3 (10.0%)	
Total not drinking	23 (95.5%)	13 (92.9%)	23 (76.7%)	54 (60.0%)
Currently drinking	1 (4.2%)	1 (7.1%)	7 (23.3%)	36 (40.0%)
Total	24	14	30	90
Men				
Life-long abstainer	1 (5.0%)	0	2 (11.1%)	
Stopped drinking	12 (60.0%)	6 (31.6%)	7 (38.9%)	
Total not drinking	13 (65.0%)	6 (31.6%)	9 (50.0%)	30 (36.0%)
Currently drinking	7 (35.0%)	13 (68.4%)	9 (50.0%)	54 (64.0%)
Total	20	19	18	84

[a] J. E. Levy and S. J. Kunitz, *Indian Drinking: Navajo Practices and Anglo-American Theories* (New York, 1974), p. 136.
[b] P. A. May and M. B. Smith, 'Some Navajo Indian Opinions about Alcohol Abuse and Prohibition', *Journal of Studies on Alcohol*, 49 (1988), pp. 324–34.

long-term (> 10 years) residents of the border town of Flagstaff, Arizona. The data are displayed in Table 6. It was striking that the prevalence of drinking was lower among Navajos than it was in nation-wide samples of the United States population, due largely to the number of people who had given up drinking. In each group sig-nificantly more men than women drank; there were significant differences among men across groups; but there were no significant differences among women across groups. A higher proportion of women in the Flagstaff and South Tuba groups were life-long abstainers than was the case in the Plateau group, but a higher proportion of women was currently drinking in Flagstaff than in the other two groups as well.

These were not weighted random samples of the Navajo population, so they cannot be combined to give estimates of the overall prevalence of drinking among Navajos in the mid-1960s. They are nonetheless useful for some comparative purposes. In 1984 May and Smith[26] surveyed the patient population of the Indian Health Service clinic in Winslow, Arizona, a border town about sixty miles east of Flagstaff, serving a large rural population adjacent to the area where our field work had been carried out eighteen years earlier. They argued that using a clinic population did not introduce significant bias into their study since every measure they had, as well as previous studies, suggested that clinic populations were indistinguishable from the larger service unit population. Their prevalence data are displayed in Table 6 along with the data from our original survey. The proportion of Navajos served by the clinic in Winslow who were currently (in 1984) not drinking (48%) was slightly higher than the estimated proportion of abstainers in the state of Arizona in 1986–8 (about 40%).[27] Most striking is the apparent increase in the prevalence of drinking among women from the mid-1960s to the mid-1980s. This is consistent with the evident increased prevalence of Fetal Alcohol Syndrome and Fetal Alcohol Effect in the Navajo population during this period as well.[28]

Changing patterns of alcohol use

In a series of papers Martin Topper has argued that as the Navajo population has grown and diversified, so have drinking styles proliferated.[29] He identifies at least five different types, several of which overlap with styles we described in our work in the 1960s and are regarded as 'traditionally' Navajo. The first type is 'the house party', which occurred at home in the evening and involved the sharing of alcoholic beverages by all adults present. The second type traditionally involved drinking by groups of older men, usually when traditional ceremonies were taking place but at a place somewhat removed from the ceremony itself. The third type was similar to the second but involved younger men. The fourth type was alcoholic drinking, which for men usually meant isolated drinking. 'The reason that his drinking was so heavily stigmatized was that it took the individual away from the economic tasks that he or she was obligated to perform and it did not involve any sharing of "drinks" among kinsmen.' On the other hand, 'The traditional female alcoholic was a person who drank in the company of men when they drank in groups in the desert or who hung around the bootlegger's house or in the trading post and traded sexual favors for liquor.'[30]

Besides these older forms of drinking have grown up new forms. 'Drinking no longer occurs more or less exclusively among kinsmen or affines. The drinking cohort often forms more or less spontaneously at various events and places.' The fact that people are not drinking with relatives and affines is disruptive, Topper argues, because the socialization function of the drinking group has vanished, and because many Navajos are suspicious of non-relatives: 'Strangers of any culture have not been easily accepted.' This difficulty relating to strangers has been exacerbated by the boarding school experience,[31] he writes, as well as by wage work, both of which are alienating and fail to meet deeply felt emotional needs.

The net impact of acculturation appears to be that only the escape of narcotizing function of alcohol remains for many young Navajos who drink in non-traditional environments. Given the fact that these people are an ever-increasing segment of the Navajo population, a major trend toward a new and dangerous form of drinking is underway. Those who drink for escape in non-traditional environments find themselves using a disinhibiting, depressant drug among strangers about whom they feel ambivalent. Furthermore, they drink in environments in which traditional Navajo rules for social control of drinking do not apply, and for which, there has not been the development of non-traditional social controls. Finally they frequently bring with them considerable anger and frustration concerning their economic and perhaps social condition. Given these factors, the increasingly high rate of alcohol-related morbidity and mortality among young Navajos is explainable. Many of these young people are neither culturally nor emotionally prepared either to tolerate the stresses of non-traditional drinking environments or to experience the emotional release or satisfaction that such drinking provides for people of other cultures. Clearly, then, these newer forms of drinking are not as therapeutic as the more traditional ones.[32]

It is important to distinguish between the causes and effects of alcohol use. We have argued that the 'traditional' patterns of alcohol use – house parties and group drinking – were not usually pathological in their causes though they were often pathological in their consequences. The new form of 'acculturated' drinking identified by Topper is more nearly pathological in its causes as well as in its consequences. He also believes that the style of acculturated drinking is becoming increasingly common and explains the increase in alcohol-related morbidity and mortality. But alcohol-related mortality seems to have decreased from the 1970s to the 1980s, which suggests there is a more complicated process at work.

We may speculate that the decline in mortality reflects the evolution of a more moderate and controlled style of drinking among people who drink for non-pathological reasons, and that the pathological drinking described by Topper has either emerged over the past generation or two or has been newly revealed by the recession of traditional drinking which may have occurred. It is not clear whether this is the case or not, but in any event it raises the important issue of 'dual diagnosis' or 'dual disorder', which has generally not been addressed in research among American Indians but which is important and related to the acculturation hypothesis. In the general population, for example, the Epidemiologic Catchment Area study[33] found that alcoholics had a 19%

lifetime rate of anxiety disorders (one and a half times the average), a 14% rate of anti-social personality (more than twenty times the average), and a 13% rate of mood disorders (nearly double the average). On the other hand, prior depression or anxiety did not raise the risk of alcoholism. It is remarkably difficult to determine whether (a) the psychiatric symptoms and the alcoholism have common causes; (b) the alcohol abuse causes acute and chronic psychiatric symptoms; or (c) psychiatric disorders produce alcohol abuse and dependence. A study of depression among the Hopi Indians of Arizona found that of forty-four individuals suffering from an affective disorder that involved depression, twelve were also diagnosed as being concurrently alcoholic or drug abusing. This included all seven males with major depression, but, without exception, the depression was secondary to their alcoholism.[34] In no case did the history of significant depression precede the onset of alcoholism or occur independent of it.

Classification

Topper's is the most elaborate typology of drinking behaviours, but there are several others. In her study of a treatment programme on the Navajo Reservation, for instance, Ferguson[35] described what she called anxiety and recreational drinkers. Both experienced the untoward consequences of alcohol use, but the recreational drinkers were older, less well educated, had more of a stake in their own society, and were much more likely to respond to the therapeutic regimen than the anxiety drinkers.[36]

Our early work was contemporaneous with Ferguson's in the mid-1960s and came to similar conclusions. In addition, we showed that many of the older men who were moderate drinkers when we interviewed them had as young men in fact experienced sequelae such as withdrawal symptoms, blackouts, accidents, and domestic and occupational troubles which all are indicators of problem drinking. And of course some men died as a result. But most men survived and either dramatically reduced or altogether ceased their drinking.[37] Young men at the time of our study were drinking in ways that were similar to what the old men had described as characteristic of their younger years. We inferred that since the drinking behaviour looked the same as what had been described historically, it was the same. Follow-up a generation later has worked to complicate the picture, as we shall describe in more detail below.

The picture for women was complicated as well. Our early work as well as Topper's subsequent typology suggested that traditionally women either drank in the protected setting of the home or they drank in the community and were considered deviants and alcoholics. Subsequently it has become evident that a higher proportion of women is drinking now than in the past, that they tend to be young, and that one of the untoward consequences is an increasing incidence of Fetal Alcohol Syndrome and Fetal Alcohol Effect. The reasons are not well understood, but it appears that as traditional sex roles are changing among Navajos – as among non-Indians – women have begun to drink in the style they have observed most commonly, in this instance in groups of peers.

Course

In considering the trajectory of alcohol use over the life course, it is usual to contrast studies of clinical and non-clinical populations.[38] There have been no formal longitudinal studies published of non-clinical Indian populations though there are observations such as ours reported immediately above which suggest that extreme drinking is common among young men in a variety of tribes and that it diminishes substantially with age. This is said to occur among the Sioux and Western Apaches in addition to the Navajos.[39]

On the other hand, there have been several studies of clinical populations. We mention only those having to do with Navajos. Savard reported that of thirty Navajo patients in an antabuse treatment programme followed for an average of nine months, 75% showed 'definite improvement'.[40] Ferguson described 115 Navajo patients followed for six months after an eighteen-month antabuse treatment period and reported a significant diminution in arrests;[41] 23% continued to be uninvolved in problem drinking at the end of the twenty-four-month period. People judged as successfully treated were older and more poorly educated than the failures.

Our own longitudinal study of Navajo alcohol use includes both clinical and non-clinical populations. It was begun in 1966 and involved interviews of four different samples of Navajo Indians, all twenty-one years of age or older. We have already described the three non-clinical populations. In addition we included a clinical population. They were thirty-five people (thirty men, five women) self-referred to the Public Health Service Indian hospital in Tuba City to be started on disulfiram in order to control their excessive alcohol consumption (called the Hospital or Antabuse group). These individuals comprised the entire population of alcohol abusers under treatment at that time.

Though we did not attempt to create an overall index of 'acculturation', the general trend was clear. The Plateau group was the least acculturated and the closest to traditional patterns. The Flagstaff group was most acculturated. The South Tuba group occupied an intermediate position. The Hospital group fell somewhere between the South Tuba and Plateau groups, reflecting the fact that approximately half of them lived in South Tuba while the rest came from areas similar to the Kaibito Plateau.

We have already described the prevalence of drinking in the three community samples. Here we describe some of the measures of amount and style of drinking.

1. Quantity–Frequency: this scale was not entirely satisfactory because much drinking in the Plateau and Hospital groups consisted of passing around a bottle of fortified wine. Estimating quantity thus was a serious problem. The South Tuba group used hard liquor and beer. The Flagstaff group used beer almost entirely and clearly distinguished their style of drinking – a beer while watching television – from the group drinking of people on Reservation, or Reservation residents who came to drink in town.

2. Definition of Alcohol: this scale was made up of statements culled from answers to the question 'What do alcoholic beverages mean to you?' The higher the score, the more likely was an individual to be a 'personal effects' rather than a social drinker. There were no significant differences among men and women across groups, which we thought may have had to do in part with the difficulty of translating some of the subtle distinctions required into Navajo. Beyond that, however, it was our impression based upon what informants told us that most people drank for similar reasons, not for oblivion or forgetfulness but to facilitate sociability.

3. Preoccupation with Alcohol: this scale measures drinking behaviour rather than motivation. It did not distinguish among women across groups, but it did not distinguish among men. The Plateau and Hospital groups described the most extreme forms of alcohol use, much more extreme than either the South Tuba or Flagstaff men. (Men and women differed only in the Plateau group.) It was also in asking these questions that we had many people tell us that alcohol had more rather than less effect on them over time; some in fact claimed that they got drunk simply by smelling a cork or open bottle of liquor. It was this observation that suggested to us that much of the drunken behaviour we saw and had reported to us was in fact learned rather than caused by true intoxication.

Data were also collected on the experience of tremulousness and hallucinations after drinking, as well as on arrest records and other social consequences of drinking. We shall not describe these findings in any detail save to say that heavy drinking resulting in withdrawal symptoms was reported most commonly by the most traditional informants.

Self-reports and life histories from our oldest informants were consistent with ethnographic reports going back into the late nineteenth century. These indicated that group drinking among young men at ceremonies was common, and those who did not wish to drink were encouraged forcibly to participate. In addition, however, since in the early years of the Reservation alcohol was expensive and hard to get, only the wealthy could afford it. A typical pattern was for a *rico* to send a rider to trade some livestock for liquor and then to dole it out to his dependants. Alcohol thus became a high prestige item of consumption.

It seemed to us that heavy drinking was the result of adherence to traditional values having to do with individual power, group solidarity, and the ability to purchase highly valued goods; that it was characteristic of young men; and that it tended to diminish very markedly as they reached their late 30s and 40s. On the other hand, drinking among women seemed to be a very different phenomenon than it was among men. A much smaller proportion of women than men used alcohol, but among those who did use alcohol there was a very high proportion who led tumultuous lives and were widely regarded as deviant in the community.

The fact that men seemed to be able to reduce their alcohol consumption as they entered early middle age was, we thought, the result of family pressure, witnessing the ravages of alcohol abuse (particularly violent deaths) among peers, and the assumption of new responsibilities as they entered a new phase of their lives. There was no doubt that alcohol use had caused serious health and family problems, and that its use had increased significantly as roads had been improved, automobiles had become more common, and Indian prohibition off Reservation ended (alcohol is still prohibited by the Tribe on Reservation). But these results led us to question the chronic addictive nature of alcohol use in this population.

Recently we have completed the analysis of follow-up interviews done in 1990 with members of the South Tuba, Plateau, and Antabuse samples (or with next of kin of those who have died) originally interviewed in 1966.[42] Our response rate has been over 99%. The results of this follow-up have complicated our initial formulations. Not surprisingly, survival analyses showed that the Hospital group had higher mortality than the other two groups, and, leaving aside the five women in that group, all the men who died, with but one exception, died of alcohol-related conditions. More surprising, the men in the Hospital group who died were on average significantly younger at the time of first interview in 1966 than those who survived (twenty-eight versus thirty-five); and they were more likely to have attended school. In addition, when the men who died were compared with men in the Hospital group who survived and are matched for age, the former were significantly younger at the time of first arrest (twenty-one versus twenty-six). There was no difference in the age at which drinking had begun; in the reported sequelae of alcohol use or in troubles due to drinking; and in arrests for assaults. Though the numbers are small, these observations suggest that there may be a stratum of heavy drinkers who are at especially high risk of premature death, and that there may be indicators early on in their drinking careers of who they may be.

The people in the Plateau and South Tuba groups who died were on average older at the time of first interview than those in the Hospital group who died, and with two exceptions they died of non-alcohol-related conditions. The net result is that when we consider all those who have survived in all three groups, they are indistinguishable in terms of age. The mean and median ages at first interview were respectively thirty-five to thirty-six and thirty-three in each of them. Twenty-three years later the survivors are on average in their late 50s.

Not only are the survivors indistinguishable in terms of age, but they are at present indistinguishable in several other important respects as well. We shall describe only three measures here: physical functioning, symptom scores of depression, and the quantity and frequency of alcohol use and of the kind of beverage consumed.

The scales of physical function are taken from the Sickness Impact Profile (SIP), which was developed in Anglo-American populations but which we have used successfully in a study of elderly Navajos.[43] This scale does not allow one to diagnose any particular disease entity. It is, rather, a way of assessing the ability to carry out normal activities of daily living (dressing, toileting, walking, and so on). The higher the score, the greater the level of disability.

The measure of depression is derived from the Center for Epidemiological Studies Depression Scale. It is a scale of symptoms commonly associated with depression. A high score is not equivalent to a clinical diagnosis of severe depression but is, rather, a measure of the severity of symptoms which may be more or less transient and situational. We have used this scale, too, in our study of the elderly.[44] It allows for estimates of one month and one year prevalence rates.

The quantity–frequency measure of alcohol use requires knowing the beverage(s) an individual consumes (in order to know their alcohol content), the amount he or she consumes, and the frequency with which it is consumed. In general, beer, wine, and liquor are the three categories of beverage. Since fortified wine is the drink of choice for many people, we have added that category as well.

First, pooling data from all the survivors, there are significant rank order correlations between most of these various scales. The SIP scales are correlated ($p < 0.001$); the two depression scales (one month and one year) are correlated ($p < 0.001$); the Body Care SIP scale is correlated with both depression scales for one month ($p < 0.005$) and one year ($p < 0.001$); age is correlated with both SIP scales ($p < 0.03$ for Body Care; $p < 0.001$ for Movement) but not with the depression scales.

Second, there is no significant difference (by Kruskal–Wallis analysis of variance) in scores of the survivors on the two scales from the SIP, either among study groups or between men and women. Nor is there a difference in the depression scale scores.

Third, there are no significant differences in the proportion of people in each group who were currently consuming alcohol at the time of follow-up. Nor were there differences in what they drank, the quantity and frequency with which they drank it, and in the proportions who considered themselves, or were considered by the interviewers, to have problems with alcohol.

Moreover, when we look back to the first interviews and ask whether there were at that time differences among members of each group who survived to 1990, the differences are not impressive. For example, Preoccupation scores of survivors (distinguishing between women and men) did not differ among groups, nor did the proportion of men who had been arrested at least once in 1961–6, nor the number of arrests for those who had been arrested. The three surviving women in the Antabuse group had all been arrested at least once in those years, but fourteen of nineteen women in the Plateau Group (73%) and nine of thirteen women in the South Tuba Group (69%) had not been. There was no significant difference in the number of arrests of those few who had been arrested (by Kruskal–Wallis analysis of variance).

These results suggest, first, that as a result of selective mortality the three groups began to look more and more alike, and second, that there existed a segment of the young male population that was at especially high risk of death from alcohol-related conditions. It is their attrition from the population that accounts for the increasing homogeneity of those who survived. This may mean that within a population where one of the traditional forms of alcohol use has been group drinking to the point of intoxication, there is a smaller population. The people in this latter group for some reason get into extremely serious difficulty with alcohol and are at high risk of premature death and are unable to moderate their use of alcohol when they reach early middle age as most Navajo men do. Based on admittedly tenuous evidence, we suspect this high-risk group may have dual diagnoses, most probably of personality disorder and alcohol abuse. If this is so, the genesis of the problems can as yet be only a matter of speculation, but it may be related to growing up in disrupted families and being sent to boarding school at a young age. Further research will be needed to test what for now must remain reasonable hypotheses.

CONCLUSIONS

The image of American Indians as people who have a great deal of trouble with alcohol has much substance behind it. But it obscures a more important reality: one characterized by heterogeneity in the past, important recent temporal changes, and diversification in the present. We think that for Navajos, the people with whom we have had most contact, the result may be both good and bad news. The good news is that the recession of the traditional patterns of the past may be contributing to the reduction in alcohol-related deaths that we have observed over the past two decades. The bad news may be that the greater proportionate importance of more pathological forms of alcohol use – if that is indeed what is occurring – may mean that treatment will be even more difficult in the future than it was in the past because a higher proportion of drinkers will be using alcohol not to enhance sociability but to treat the symptoms, or as a manifestation, of psychopathology. If that is true – and only future research will determine if it is – then not only will the treatment system be challenged in new ways, but new kinds of preventive efforts and early interventions will have to be designed as well.

NOTES

1 Alcohol-related deaths include deaths due to alcoholism, alcoholic psychoses, and cirrhosis of the liver with mention of alcoholism. Source: Indian Health Service, *Trends in Indian Health 1991* (Washington, DC: US Department of Health and Human Services, Public Health Service, 1991).
2 For useful surveys see, D. B. Heath, 'Alcohol Use among North American Indians: A Cross-Cultural Survey of Patterns and Problems', in R. G. Smart *et al.*, eds., *Research Advances in Alcohol and Drug Problems* (New York, 1983), and P. A. May, 'Explanations of Native American Drinking: A Literature Review', *Plains Anthropologist*, 22 (1977), 223–32.
3 P. May, 'Alcohol Abuse and Alcoholism among American Indians: An Over-

view', in T. D. Watts and R. Wright, Jr, eds., *Alcoholism in Minority Populations* (Springfield, 1989), pp. 100–1.

4 See, for example, R. Jessor, T. D. Graves, R. C. Hanson, and S. L. Jessor, *Society, Personality, and Deviant Behavior: A Study of a Tri-Ethnic Community* (New York, 1968), and T. D. Graves, 'Acculturation, Access, and Alcohol in a Tri-Ethnic Community', *American Anthropologist*, 69 (1967), 306–21.

5 C. MacAndrew and R. B. Edgerton, *Drunken Comportment: A Social Explanation* (Chicago, 1969).

6 J. E. Levy and S. J. Kunitz, *Indian Drinking: Navajo Practices and Anglo-American Theories* (New York, 1974). See also J. Leland, *Firewater Myths* (New Brunswick, N.J.: Rutgers Center of Alcohol Studies, 1976).

7 Levy and Kunitz, *Indian Drinking*.

8 The data are from the following publication: Indian Health Service, *Regional Differences in Indian Health, 1991* (Washington, DC: US Department of Health and Human Services, Public Health Service, 1991). Evidently in three of the areas there have been problems with listing the decedents' race as Indian. These areas are Oklahoma, California, and Portland. The result seems to be that the reported rates are lower than the real rates.

9 The data are from the following publication: Indian Health Service, *Selected Vital Statistics for Indian Health Service Areas and Service Units, 1972 to 1977*, DHEW Publication No. (HSA) 79–1005 (Rockville, Md.: US Department of Health and Human Services, Public Health Service, 1979). Because people may leave their service units of residence and die elsewhere, they may not be counted in their service unit rates. Thus the rates reported are for the resident population. As we shall indicate, emigration can result in substantial under-reporting of deaths.

10 K. M. Stewart, 'Yumans: Introduction', in A. Ortiz, ed., *Handbook of North American Indians, Vol. 10, Southwest* (Washington, DC: Smithsonian Institution, 1983), p. 2.

11 R. Stratton, A. Zeiner, and A. Paredes, 'Tribal Affiliation and Prevalence of Alcohol Problems', *Journal of Studies on Alcohol*, 39 (1978), 1166–77. See also R. Stratton, 'Relationship between Prevalence of Alcohol Problems and Socio-economic Conditions among Oklahoma Native Americans', *Currents in Alcoholism*, 8 (1981), 315–25.

12 P. A. May, K. J. Hymbaugh, J. M. Aase, and J. M. Samet, 'Epidemiology of fetal alcohol syndrome among American Indians of the Southwest', *Social Biology*, 30 (1983), 374–87.

13 The Hopi data appear in J. E. Levy, S. J. Kunitz, and E. Henderson, 'Hopi Deviance in Historical and Epidemiological Perspective', in L. Donald, ed., *Themes in Ethnology and Culture History* (Berkeley, Calif., Folklore Institute, 1987). The Navajo data are from Indian Health Service, *Indian Health Trends and Services 1970 Edition* (Rockville, Md.: PHS Publication No. 2092, Office of Program Planning and Evaluation, Program Analysis and Statistics Branch, Indian Health Service, US Department of Health, Education and Welfare, 1971), and S. J. Kunitz, *Disease Change and the Role of Medicine: The Navajo Experience* (Berkeley, Calif., 1983).

14 Space limitations do not permit a discussion of the problems involved in arriving at these rates. We believe the true average annual rate probably lies somewhere between 7 and 14 per 100,000 in the mid-1960s.

15 Kunitz, *Disease Change*, p. 104.

16 Levy and Kunitz, *Indian Drinking*.

17 B. F. Grant, T. S. Zobeck, and R. P. Pickering, *Liver Cirrhosis Mortality in the United States, 1973–87*, Surveillance report no. 15 (Rockville, Md.: National Institute on Alcohol Abuse and Alcoholism, Division of Biometry and Epidemiology, Alcohol Epidemiologic Data System, US Department of Health and Human Services, 1991).

18 Kunitz, *Disease Change*, p. 104.

19 The cirrhosis rates in 1985–8 are calculated for ICDA 9 codes 571.0, 571.1, 571.2, and 571.3, all alcohol-related. If codes 571.5 and 571.6 are added, the rates for men are 13.9–15.8, and for women 10.0–11.4.

20 Kunitz, *Disease Change*, pp. 101–2.

21 T. S. Zobeck, S. D. Elliott, B. F. Grant, and D. Bertolucci. *Trends in Alcohol-Related Fatal Traffic Crashes, United States: 1977–88*, Surveillance report no. 17 (Rockville, Md.: National Institute on Alcohol Abuse and Alcoholism, Division of Biometry and Epidemiology, Alcohol Epidemiologic Data System, US Department of Health and Human Services, 1991).

22 P. S. Katz and P. A. May, *Motor Vehicle Accidents on the Navajo Reservation 1973–75* (Window Rock, Ariz.: Navajo Health Authority, 1979).

23 *Ibid.*, p. 65.

24 The Indian Health Service assumes that 60% of motor vehicle accident deaths are alcohol related (Navajo Area Indian Health Service, *Health Statistics Report: Alcohol-Related Mortality/Morbidity and Violence* (Window Rock, Ariz.: Office of Program Planning and Development, NAIHS, US Public Health Service 1990).

25 Levy and Kunitz, *Indian Drinking*.

26 P. A. May and M. B. Smith, 'Some Navajo Indian Opinions about Alcohol Abuse and Prohibition: A Survey and Recommendations for Policy', *Journal of Studies on Alcohol*, 49 (1988), 324–34.

27 G. D. Williams, F. S. Stinson, S. D. Brooks, and J. Noble, *Apparent per Capita Alcohol Consumption: National, State and Regional Trends: 1977–88* (Rockville, Md.: National Institute on Alcohol Abuse and Alcoholism, Division of Biometry and Epidemiology, Alcohol Epidemiologic Data System, US Department of Health and Human Services, 1991), p. 36.

28 May *et al.*, 'Epidemiology of fetal alcohol syndrome'.

29 M. D. Topper, 'Navajo "alcoholism": Drinking, Alcohol Abuse, and Treatment in a Changing Cultural Environment', in L. Bennett and G. Ames, eds., *The American Experience with Alcohol: Contrasting Cultural Perspectives* (New York, 1985). M. D. Topper and J. Curtis, 'Extended Family Therapy: A Clinical Approach to the Treatment of Synergistic Dual Anomic Depression among Navajo Agency-Town Adolescents', *Journal of Community Psychology*, 15 (1987), 334–48.

30 Topper, 'Navajo "alcoholism"', pp. 232–5.

31 It has been a policy since the nineteenth century to send Navajo and other Indian youngsters away to boarding schools. Originally the schools were run by church groups, more recently by the Bureau of Indian Affairs, part of the Department of the Interior of the federal government. The object was to take children from their homes and teach them to be Anglo-Americans. Boarding

schools have fallen into increasing disrepute in recent years, and a decreasing proportion of students attend them. Most now attend day schools in or near their home communities. It is thought that as a result, the youngsters being sent to boarding schools are likely to be from troubled homes, and are themselves especially likely to have emotional and psychological difficulties.

32 Topper, 'Navajo "alcoholism"', pp. 238–9.

33 D. A. Regier *et al.*, 'Comorbidity of Mental Disorders with Alcohol and Other Drug Abuse: Results from the Epidemiologic Catchment (ECA) Study', *Journal of the American Medical Association*, 264 (1990), 2511–18.

34 S. M. Manson, J. H. Shore, and J. D. Bloom, 'The Depressive Experience in American Indian Communities: A Challenge for Psychiatric Theory and Diagnosis', in A. Kleinman and B. Good, eds., *Culture and Depression: Studies in the Anthropology and Cross-Cultural Psychiatry of Affective Disorder* (Berkeley, Calif., 1985).

35 F. N. Ferguson, 'Navajo Drinking: Some Tentative Hypotheses', *Human Organization*, 27 (1968), 159–67; and 'A Treatment Program for Navajo Alcoholics: Results after Four Years', *Quarterly Journal of Studies on Alcohol*, 31 (1970), 898–919.

36 F. N. Ferguson, 'Stake Theory as an Explanatory Device in Navajo Alcoholism Treatment Response', *Human Organization*, 35 (1976), 65–78.

37 Levy and Kunitz, *Indian Drinking*.

38 K. M. Fillmore, *Alcohol Use Across the Life Course: A Critical Review of 70 Years of International Longitudinal Research* (Toronto: Addiction Research Foundation, 1988).

39 T. W. Hill, 'From Hell-Raiser to Family Man', in J. Spradley and D. McCurdy, eds., *Conformity and Conflict: Readings in Cultural Anthropology*, 2nd edn (Boston, 1974).

40 R. J. Savard, 'Effects of Disulfiram Therapy on Relationships within the Navajo Drinking Group', *Quarterly Journal of Studies on Alcohol*, 29 (1968), 909–16.

41 Ferguson, 'Navajo Drinking', and 'A Treatment Program for Navajo Alcoholics'.

42 S. J. Kunitz and J. E. Levy, 'Drinking Careers. A Twenty-Five Year Follow-up of Three Navajo Populations' (New Haven, 1994).

43 S. J. Kunitz and J. E. Levy, *Navajo Aging: From Family to Institutional Support* (Tucson, 1991).

44 *Ibid.*, ch. 4.

EIGHT

THE DRUG HABIT: THE ASSOCIATION OF THE WORD 'DRUG' WITH ABUSE IN AMERICAN HISTORY

JOHN PARASCANDOLA

WHAT kind of image does the term 'drug user' generally bring to mind in today's society? Is the average response to a statement that someone is 'taking drugs' likely to be an inquiry about what type of illness he or she is suffering from and what medication is being used to treat it? Probably not, because for most people 'taking drugs' tends to have a connotation that links it with abuse rather than with medicinal use.

Yet the word 'drug' was not always so closely linked in the public mind with substance abuse. The definition of the noun drug in volume III (published in 1897) of the original edition of the *Oxford English Dictionary* (OED) is as follows: 'An original, simple medicinal substance, organic or inorganic, whether used by itself in its natural condition or prepared by art, or as an ingredient in a medicine or medicament.'[1]

The OED went on to discuss other aspects of the history and use of the term that need not be considered here. From the point of view of this essay, the key fact to note is that the noun drug is associated with medicinal or related use. There is no reference to recreational use or abuse of a substance in the definition.

The first edition of the OED was not completed until 1928, and the first supplement, providing the earliest opportunity to modify a definition already in print, was not published until 1933. That supplementary volume, however, adds a new definition for the noun drug, in addition to the traditional one already quoted. The addition reads as follows: 'Now often applied without qualification to narcotics and opiates.' Drug addict, drug evil, drug fiend, and drug habit are given as examples of this usage.[2]

This essay will focus on the evolution of this latter use of the word drug in the United States and on the effort by American pharmacists in the 1920s to combat this trend, a battle that they obviously lost as evidenced by the use of the term today. The association of the term drug with substance abuse appears to have had its beginnings at the very end of the nineteenth century. In attempting to track down the earliest uses of the word in this sense in the medical literature, a good place to begin is with *Index Medicus*, the monthly guide to the world's medical periodical literature established by John Shaw Billings in 1879.[3] The only subject heading related to substance abuse in the first four volumes of *Index Medicus* is 'Alcoholism', which appears as a subheading under 'Diseases of the Nervous System'. By the fifth volume, in 1883, the heading was expanded to 'Alcoholism and Opium Habit', which soon became 'Alcoholism, Opium Habit, etc.'. The 'etc.' reflects the increasing literature on other habit-forming drugs, such as tobacco and cocaine.

An analysis of the titles of the articles listed under these headings, however, did not reveal a single one that referred to the drug habit, drug addiction, or some similar designation in the early years of publication of *Index Medicus*. Mostly these publications were concerned with specific individual habits, such as alcoholism or morphinism. The first reference to 'drug habits' in a more generic sense in the title of an article appeared in 1897, coincidentally the same year in which the OED volume with its traditional definition of the word drug was published.[4] After that year, one begins to see several articles a year that use such terms or phrases as drug habits, drug habitués, drug patients, drug addiction, and abuse of drugs in their titles.

All of these articles through the year 1907 were published in American journals. There would appear to be no reference in *Index Medicus* to this use of the word drug (or its counterpart in a foreign language) in the title of an article published outside the United States before 1908, in spite of the international coverage of the publication. In 1908, a South African medical journal published an article that referred to drug habits in its title.[5] Of course, this does not mean that the term drug was never used in such a way in other countries during this period. The term 'drug habits' was used in the body of the text of a British publication in 1903, for example, and no doubt there are other cases to be found of the use of this term and similar ones.[6] Yet if one can assume that use of a word in the title of publications is some measure of its popularity, then the evidence from *Index Medicus* suggests, at least with respect to the medical literature, that this form of usage first became common in the United States.

Even in the United States, however, the association of the word drug with abuse does not seem to have gained widespread usage until about the time of the First World War, or shortly before. For example, drug habit does not appear as a term in the index of *Index Medicus* until 1916, and even then only as a cross-reference to 'narcotic habit' (which had come to replace the old 'opium habit'). Three years later, drug habit became a main entry in the index.[7] Similarly, drug habit does not appear as a subject heading in the *Index-Catalogue* of the Surgeon General's Library until the third series, in the volume published in 1923.[8] The volume that included the letter 'D' in the second series had been published in 1899, so the term could not have been added between then and 1923.

That this usage of the word drug may have become more widespread in the popular as well as the medical literature around the time of the First World War is suggested by the fact that drug habit first appeared as a subject heading in the *Reader's Guide to Periodical Literature* in the third volume, published in 1915 and covering the literature for 1910 through 1914.[9] The first issue of the *New York Times* index, published in January 1913, already included drug evil as a subject heading.[10] In the *Encyclopedia Britannica*, an influential popular reference tool in the United States as well as in Britain, the term drug does not appear as an entry until the eleventh edition, published in 1910. In addition to discussing the word in a medical sense, the *Britannica* goes on to add: 'In a particular sense "drug" is often used synonymously for narcotics or poisonous substances, and hence "to drug" means to stupefy or poison.'[11] Thus by 1910 the term drug was commonly enough equated with narcotic to merit mention of this fact in the most noted English-language encyclopedia.

Why did this switch from a consistent reference to specific problems such as opium habit to a more generic reference to the drug habit take place in this period? It is difficult to give a definitive answer to this question, but we can at least identify some of the likely factors involved.

The statement quoted above from the *Encyclopedia Britannica* suggests one of the sources for this meaning. Although the noun drug was apparently not commonly used in place of such terms as narcotic in designating abuse or addiction before about the turn of this century, the verb drug has a long history of association with attempts to stupefy or poison someone, the use noted in the *Britannica* definition. The OED in 1897 gives two definitions for the verb drug that are related to narcotics: (1) to mix or adulterate food or drink with a drug, especially a narcotic or poisonous drug; (2) to administer drugs to a person, especially for the purpose of stupefying or poisoning him. The earliest reference they give for either of these related meanings is to Shakespeare's *Macbeth* in 1605, where the phrase 'I have drugged their Possets' appears.[12]

That the use of drug to mean narcotic was derived, or at least gained credence from, this older usage of the verb is supported by the following

THE NEW YORK TIMES, SUNDAY, NOVEMBER 9, 1924.

ONE MILLION AMERICANS VICTIMS OF DRUG HABIT

Alarming Increase of Addicts Called Menace More Dangerous Than War—U. S. Now Consumes Four Times as
Much as All Europe—Youth the Victim

This *New York Times* headline from 1924 exemplified the common use of
the term drug to designate narcotics and similar substances. (With the
permission of the *New York Times*.)

quotation from an American pharmaceutical journal of the 1920s
commenting on the practice: 'It may be true, as has been contended by
defenders of the practice, that the use of "drug" in the sense of
"stupefy" is long established and that it is found in classical literature
and has had the sanction of the best writers.'[13]

Given this long association of the verb drug with the administration
of narcotics or poisons, it is not surprising that the noun drug should
come to be used by many synonymously with narcotics or like substances. It is perhaps more puzzling to contemplate why such usage
apparently did not begin to become common before the end of the
nineteenth century.

One of the answers to this question is suggested by an examination of
the medical literature of the period. As the 1880s and 1890s progressed,
the number of substances that attracted the attention of the medical
community because of their potential to induce a habit increased well
beyond the traditional opium and alcohol. The use of the term 'etc.' in
the subject heading in *Index Medicus* has already been mentioned as an
example of the increasing diversity of drugs cited in the articles covered.
A search of titles listed in *Index Medicus* in the 1880s and early 1890s
reveals articles dealing with a host of abused substances, including
opium, morphine, alcohol, tobacco, cocaine, ether, coffee, absinthe,
chloral, hashish, antifebrin, and paraldehyde. Physicians were no
doubt struggling for some term that could link all of these substance
abuse problems together, that could cover the generic problem. In fact,
one can clearly see the efforts to do this by the use of such terms as
voluntary intoxications, diseased cravings, and morbid longings in the
titles of articles in this period.[14] Once the term drug habit (or habits)
was introduced, one can see why it might have appealed to many of the
more scientifically minded physicians as being more exact and less

judgemental than references to morbid and diseased cravings and longings. Although the lay public may have been less worried about such
niceties, terms such as drug habit and drug evil (with its more negative
connotation) still probably seemed to be useful and simple general
designations, a convenient shorthand, for what was perceived as a
growing problem.

Certainly there was increasing concern about drug abuse on the part
of the American medical profession and the public in the late nineteenth and early twentieth centuries. The evidence suggests that opiate
addiction was on the rise in the United States between the end of the
Civil War and the close of the century. Even after the rate apparently
began to decline somewhere around 1900, government and private
statistics of the day tended greatly to overestimate the number of
addicts. In addition, as various historians have pointed out, the image
of the addict changed, from that of a middle-class victim accidentally
addicted through medicinal use to that of a criminal or otherwise
deviant individual who had turned to drugs for purely recreational
reasons. Public fear of this abuse was thus heightened.[15]

Various reformers waged a vigorous campaign against the evils of
addiction to narcotics and other drugs, leading to the passage of the
Harrison Narcotics Act in 1914 and then to strict interpretation of the
Act to deny physicians the right to maintain the habits of existing
addicts. In the course of this campaign, the public was frequently
exposed to newspaper headlines and stories in popular magazines about
the drug evil and drug fiends.[16] Sometimes the slang term 'dope' was
used to designate abused substances in the popular literature, but drug
all too often became a synonym for dope. And in the medical literature
of the period, it was the term of choice to denote the generic problem,
since dope was hardly a scientific word.

By the 1920s, some American pharmacists had become concerned
enough about the growing negative connotation of the word drug to
urge that steps should be taken to correct the problem. Since pharmacies were more commonly known as drugstores, the pharmacists as
druggists, in the United States at that time, it is understandable that the
profession was worried about the public's image of drugs. This concern
was heightened by the fact that occasional scandals linked certain
pharmacists and drug stores with the illegal sale of narcotics.[17] In
addition, under the recently enacted Prohibition Amendment, pharmacies were the major legal suppliers of liquor, and some in the
profession feared the negative image that this situation might create in
the public mind, especially if too many of their colleagues filled what
one druggist referred to as ' "camouflage" prescriptions'.[18]

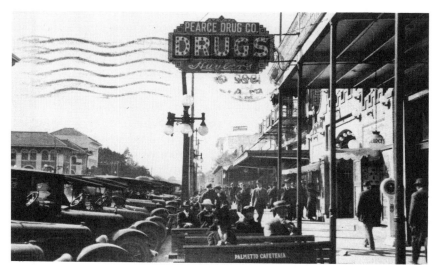

This 1920s Florida drugstore, as depicted on a postcard, displays the large 'Drugs' sign typical of American pharmacies. Many pharmacists of the period were concerned about the increasing identification of the word drug with abuse. (Courtesy of William H. Helfand.)

One prominent pharmacy leader of the period who seems to have waged his own private war against the misuse of the term drug was Dr Edward Kremers, head of the pharmacy programme at the University of Wisconsin.[19] After receiving his undergraduate education in pharmacy and science at the University of Wisconsin in Madison, Kremers had then gone on to Germany to pursue graduate work in chemistry. He obtained his doctoral degree from the University of Göttingen in 1890. Upon his return to the United States, he joined the faculty of the department of pharmacy at Wisconsin, succeeding to the chair in 1892.

By the 1920s, Kremers was well established as a reformer in American pharmaceutical education. At this time, he began writing to the editors of various publications when he saw them using the word drug instead of narcotic or a similar term. For example, in 1923, he wrote to the Narcotic Education Association about a booklet they published on the opium problem, which was described as being a 'scientific' treatment of the subject. Kremers asked: 'If the treatise is scientifically exact, why do you speak of the "drug habit." Not all drugs are habit forming drugs. The misuse of the term drug in recent years is bringing all drugs into disrepute.'[20]

Similarly, he complained to the editor of *The Nation* in 1929 about an article appearing in that publication: 'As a pharmacist, I resent the loose usage of the term drug. It is not synonymous with narcotic. For every narcotic drug – using the term in a modern legal sense – there are a hundred, if not a thousand drugs not subject to narcotic legislation.'[21]

Kremers, incidentally, did not just attack the misuse of the word drug in his letters to editors. Frequently he also challenged the general views of some of the anti-narcotic forces. He himself did not believe that prohibition of narcotics would be any more successful in curbing their use than prohibition of alcohol seemed to him to be slowing the consumption of alcohol in the 1920s. Even if all the opium plants in the world could be destroyed, and Kremers pointed out that the drug had its legitimate therapeutic uses, he felt that methods for producing synthetic drugs in small laboratories would be developed to meet the demand. He was also angered by the tendency of many of the anti-drug crusaders to blame the problem on foreigners, when in his view those Americans whose greed drove them to sell illicit drugs were really more responsible for the situation.[22]

Perhaps the first organized effort by professional pharmacy to combat the misuse of the term drug was initiated by the journal *Pacific Drug Review*. In March 1922, the journal announced that the widespread use of the term drug to mean narcotic had prompted it to institute a campaign to combat this practice. The editors of the publication sent letters about this issue to pharmacists, newspaper editors, politicians, and others to urge their cooperation in the effort to distinguish between the legitimate and illegitimate use of drugs. In the pages of the journal, they urged every pharmacist to become a 'committee of one' to take up the subject with the editor of his or her local newspaper, as they were convinced that the press was the chief offender. *Pacific Drug Review* reprinted newspaper headlines illustrating the offending practices, and noted that thanks to the press the public was coming to associate the 'drug trade' with a criminal activity.[23]

Another manifestation of the concern of pharmacists about the misuse of the term drug in the 1920s was a campaign initiated by the Drug Trade Board of Public Information, a public relations organization on behalf of the pharmaceutical trade established in 1920. The Board consisted of representatives of eight national pharmaceutical associations, representing various aspects of the field from retail pharmacists to wholesale druggists to manufacturers.[24] Its director was Robert P. Fischelis, who was lecturer in commercial pharmacy at the Philadelphia College of Pharmacy and also had a consulting office in New York. Fischelis soon thereafter became dean of the New Jersey College of Pharmacy and went on to have a distinguished career in pharmacy.[25]

In June of 1922, the Board addressed an appeal to 500 newspapers around the country, enlisting their support in an effort to curb the misuse of the word drug in connection with stories involving the illegal use of narcotics. The appeal was released as a 'bulletin' from the Board's News Service, and was in the form of a letter from Fischelis addressed to the managing editors of the newspapers, 'not necessarily for publication, but rather for the information of your editorial staff'. The newspapers were reminded that the term drug included all substances used in the cure or mitigation of disease, of which narcotic substances represented only a small portion, and even then their medicinal use was tightly controlled. Editors and reporters were urged to refer to narcotics or narcotic drugs in stories dealing with narcotics or 'dope'. Headlines such as 'Drug Peddlers Held in Raid' were damaging to the legitimate drug trade. Fischelis noted:

We believe that you can readily understand that the use of the word 'drug,' which covers a legitimate field of activity, in describing something illegitimate, reacts to the detriment of the legitimate portion of the industry . . . It is therefore manifestly unfair to stigmatize this industry by the mis-use of the word 'drug.' The public at once begins to associate any kind of drug with dope or narcotics and naturally associates dope peddlers with people in the drug business.[26]

The Drug Trade Board's effort was given wider publicity within the pharmaceutical profession when its appeal to newspapers was reprinted in *American Druggist and Pharmaceutical Record* in July of 1922.[27]

The issue of misuse of the word drug was also a topic of concern at the 1922 meeting of the National Association of Retail Druggists (NARD), one of the affiliated members of the Drug Trade Board, held in Detroit that September. NARD is an organization of drug store owners, not all of whom are registered pharmacists. In his presidential address, Ambrose Hunsberger mentioned that efforts were being made (presumably those previously discussed) to convince newspapers to use the qualifying term 'narcotic' whenever using the word 'drug' to mean a narcotic, or to substitute the slang term 'dope' for drug. He told his audience:

This campaign has met with success in some instances and in others objection was raised to the qualifying term 'narcotic' as being too long for headline use, and to the word 'dope' because of the fact that it is slang. The latter objection seems unwarranted in the light of the language that appears in most of the newspapers of the day and it is suggested that our members take advantage of every opportunity to encourage their local newspapers to make use of the qualifying term or the word 'dope.' Constant usage will eventually add this word to our language, rendering the use of a confusing term unnecessary.[28]

The Association's Committee on Public relations also bemoaned the harm done to the industry by this misuse of the term drug in its report at the meeting. The Committee optimistically and somewhat naively claimed that this misuse would be entirely eliminated 'if the public knew that the word "Drug" is as applicable to quinine as it is to cocaine'.[29]

One of those attending the meeting was Charles H. Eyles, president of the Richard A. Foley Advertising Agency in Philadelphia. The agency represented Johnson & Johnson, many of whose products were marketed in drug stores. At the time, the Foley Advertising Agency was already conducting a campaign for Johnson & Johnson in support of the image of the pharmacist, involving the slogan 'Your Druggist is More Than a Merchant – Try the Drug Store First'. Eyles apparently convinced Johnson & Johnson to support the effort to correct the misuse of the word drug.

Eyles wrote to some 400 newspapers and magazines, enclosing a copy of an editorial from the July 1922 issue of *American Druggist* that explained the case for not using drug to mean narcotic, and asked the publishers for their consideration in this matter. Eyles claimed that in general he received cooperative response, and that many publications reprinted the *American Druggist* editorial or published one of their own along similar lines. If one can judge from the excerpts from replies that he included in a brochure on the subject, however, it would appear that what he called 'letters of endorsement and cooperation' were often rather non-committal. While *The Sacramento Bee* informed Eyles that they already had such a policy in place, the more common responses cited were along the lines of: I have read your letter carefully and communicated it verbally to the editorial staff; it will probably take a long time to break the habit of using the term in this way; the modern drug store is very important; we are very interested in this subject and have spent considerable energy helping in the fight against 'dope'. Since it was obviously in Eyles' best interest to demonstrate how successful his campaign had been, it is reasonable to assume that these responses were among the more positive responses that he had received.[30]

Eyles' self-congratulatory brochure on the campaign, perhaps issued as much to publicize his advertising agency as to help further the effort, claimed that the problem was being corrected, in part as a result of this campaign. Yet the evidence suggests that the campaign did little if anything to reverse the use of the word drug in connection with illegal use of narcotics and other abused substances. Drug habit, drug fiend, drug traffic and the like continued to be commonly used by the press.[31]

The 1920s campaign on the part of the American pharmaceutical profession to curb what pharmacists saw as misuse of the term drug appears to have died a quiet death within a few short years. In what was perhaps a last-gasp effort, the American Pharmaceutical Association passed a resolution at its annual meeting in 1930 to urge newspapers to use 'the words "narcotic" or "narcotic drug" in the place of the designation "drug" when narcotics are referred to in the news of the day'.[32]

It is obvious from our perspective today, of course, that pharmacists lost the battle. Their belief that they could educate the public about the 'correct' use of the word and disassociate it from substance abuse was naive and overly optimistic. Pharmacists today, as well as the rest of the public, still have to live with the dual meaning of the term. There have been efforts from some factions in pharmacy to deal with the problem in a different way, namely to try to substitute a different term for drug in therapeutic contexts. For example, a 1987 list of standard terminology issued by the American Pharmaceutical Association urged pharmacists to use the terms 'medicine' and 'medication' and to avoid using drug 'when therapeutic qualities are to be highlighted'.[33]

In its 1974 report on *Drug Use in America*, the National Commission on Marihuana and Drug Abuse drew a clear and useful distinction between the use of the word drug in the therapeutic and in the social context. In the social sense, the Commission pointed out, drug is not a neutral term, but has a value component reflected in phrases such as 'drug problem'.[34] We would not be likely to have any more success than the pharmacists of the 1920s if we attempted to reverse this trend. We can only be careful to specify the context in which we use the term, and to recognize the connotations surrounding such use.

NOTES

1 James A. H. Murray, Henry Bradley, William A. Craigie, and C. T. Onions, eds., *A New English Dictionary on Historical Principles*, 10 vols. (Oxford, 1888–1928), III (pt I) (1897), first p. 687.

2 W. A. Craigie and C. T. Onions, *Introduction, Supplement and Bibliography* (to ibid.) (Oxford, 1933), first p. 309.

3 On the origins and history of *Index Medicus*, see John B. Blake, ed., *Centenary of Index Medicus, 1879–1979* (Bethesda, Md., 1979). See also the introductory material in *Index Medicus*, 1 (1897), pp. 1–28, for information on the purpose and methodology of the publication and a list of the original journals indexed.

4 *Index Medicus*, 20 (1897), p. 153. The citation is to F. X. Dercum, 'The Drug Habits', in H. A. Hare, ed., *A System of Practical Therapeutics*, 4 vols. (Philadelphia, 1891–7), IV (1897), pp. 795–817. I am aware of at least one earlier reference that I did not find cited in *Index Medicus*. See Carl Frese, 'Drug-

Habits', in J. C. Wilson, ed., *An American Text-Book of Applied Therapeutics for the Use of Practitioners and Students* (Philadelphia, 1896), pp. 59–72.

5 *Index Medicus*, 2nd series 6 (1908), p. 428. The citation is to C. McC. Kitching, 'Treatment of Drug Habits as Illustrated by that of Opium and Morphine', *South African Medical Record*, 6 (1908), pp. 33–5.

6 Henry Campbell, 'The Study of Inebriety: A Retrospect and a Forecast', *British Journal of Inebriety* 1 (1903), pp. 5–14, see p. 11.

7 'Index of Subjects', *Index Medicus*, 2nd series 14 (1916), p. 96; *ibid.*, 2nd series 17 (1919), p. 118.

8 *Index-Catalogue of the Library of the Surgeon General's Office, United States Army*, 3rd series, 10 vols. (Washington, DC, 1918–32), IV (1923), pp. 736–41.

9 *Readers' Guide to Periodical Literature [Cumulated]*, III (New York, 1910–14; published 1915), p. 762.

10 *The New York Times Index*, vol. 1, no. 1, Jan.–Mar. 1913 (New York, 1965 (reprint)), p. 64.

11 *Encyclopedia Britannica*, 11th edn, 29 vols. (New York, 1910), VII, p. 597.

12 See n. 1.

13 '"Drugs" and "Narcotics"', *Pacific Drug Review*, 34 [3] (March 1922), p. 9.

14 See, e.g., *Index Medicus*, 11 (1889), p. 359; *ibid.*, 12 (1890), p. 329; *ibid.*, 14 (1892), p. 14.

15 For discussions of the number and perception of drug addicts in the United States in this period, see David F. Musto, *The American Disease: Origins of Narcotic Control*, expanded edition (New York, 1987); David T. Courtwright, *Dark Paradise: Opiate Addiction in America before 1940* (Cambridge, Mass., 1982); H. Wayne Morgan, *Drugs in America: A Social History, 1800–1980* (Syracuse, 1981).

16 For a significant sampling of this type of story in newspapers and popular magazines, see Gary Silver, ed., *The Dope Chronicles, 1850–1950* (San Francisco, 1979), which consists largely of reproductions of newspaper and magazine clippings. See also such previously cited indexes to the newspaper and magazine literature such as *Readers' Guide* and *New York Times Index*.

17 Courtwright, *Dark Paradise*, pp. 51–2; Morgan, *Drugs*, p. 102.

18 See, e.g., 'Shall We Be Liquor Dealers?', *American Druggist*, 69 (1921), p. 40.

19 On Kremers, see George Urdang, 'Edward Kremers (1865–1941): Reformer of American Pharmaceutical Education', *American Journal of Pharmaceutical Education*, 11 (1947), pp. 631–58.

20 Copy of letter from Edward Kremers to Narcotic Education Association, 31 March 1923, Kremers Reference Files (hereafter referred to as KRF), c46(i)1: United States, F. B. Power Pharmaceutical Library, University of Wisconsin–Madison.

21 Copy of letter from Edward Kremers to Editor of *The Nation*, 3 May 1929, KRF, c46(i)1: United States.

22 See, e.g., *ibid.*; copies of letters from Edward Kremers to Editor of *Dearborn Independent*, 10 April 1924, and to Narcotic Education Association, 13 April 1923, KRF, c46(i)1: United States.

23 '"Drugs" and "Narcotics"', *Pacific Drug Review*, 34 [3] (March 1922), p. 9; 'Say "Narcotic", Rather than "Drug"', *ibid.*, pp. 16–19.

24 'Drug Trade Board of Public Information', *American Druggist*, 68 [4] (April

1920), p. 70; 'Eight National Associations Maintain a Board for Informing the Public', *Druggists Circular*, 66 [4] (April 1922), p. 148; 'Drug Trade Bureau of Public Information', *American Druggist*, 71 [2] (February 1923), p. 24.

25 On Fischelis, see Roy A. Bowers and David L. Cowen, *The Rutgers University College of Pharmacy: A Centennial History* (New Brunswick, N.J., 1991), pp. 220–1; Joseph W. England, ed., *The First Century of the Philadelphia College of Pharmacy 1821–1921* (Philadelphia, 1922), pp. 427–8.

26 Unnumbered and undated bulletin from the News Service of the Drug Trade Board of Public Information addressed from Robert Fischelis 'To the Managing Editor', box on Drug Trade Bureau of Public Information, American Pharmaceutical Association Archives, Washington, DC. The date of June 1922 was deduced from the published reference to this bulletin cited in n. 27. I am indebted to George Griffenhagen for locating and providing me with a copy of this document and the bulletin cited in n. 32.

27 'Newspapers Urged to Discontinue Misuse of Term "Drug"', *American Druggist*, 70 [7] (July 1922), p. 43.

28 Ambrose Hunsberger, 'President's Address', *N.A.R.D. Journal*, 35 (1922), pp. 54–9; the quotation is from pp. 55–6.

29 'Report of the Committee on Public Relations', *N.A.R.D. Journal*, 35 (1922), pp. 98–9; the quotation is from p. 98.

30 'Correcting Misuse of the Word "Drug"', p. 14, undated promotional booklet published by the Richard A. Foley Advertising Agency, Philadelphia, copy in KRF, c34(d)1: Drug Nomenclature.

31 See n. 16.

32 *Journal of the American Pharmaceutical Association*, 19 (1930), p. 526. See also bulletin 1930–12 from the Drug Trade Bureau of Public Information, 29 May 1930, box on Drug Trade Bureau of Public Information, American Pharmaceutical Association Archives, Washington, DC.

33 George B. Griffenhagen, memorandum on 'APhA Standard Terminology', 1 January 1987, copy in possession of author. I am indebted to Michael Harris and George Griffenhagen for this memo.

34 National Commission on Marihuana and Drug Use, *Drug Use in America: Problem in Perspective* (New York, 1974), p. 9.

NINE

RESEARCH AND DEVELOPMENT IN THE UK PHARMACEUTICAL INDUSTRY FROM THE NINETEENTH CENTURY TO THE 1960S

JUDY SLINN

INTRODUCTION

SUCCESS in the international pharmaceutical industry today is built on the discovery of new and better drugs for the treatment and cure of disease and their introduction to markets across the world. New drugs must be sold worldwide, since no company can fully exploit a patented product, recouping its research and development costs solely in its own home market, even in the two largest national markets, the USA and Japan. The ability of any company to innovate successfully largely depends on its resources although there is also an element of serendipity in the discovery of new drugs. Successful penetration of world markets depends on the product and its skilful marketing to secure maximum returns which, in turn, will finance further research and development.

The history of the British pharmaceutical industry and the growth of its research and development capability, to take a not insignificant place in the international industry in the late twentieth century, can conveniently be considered in three periods since the late nineteenth century. The divisions are marked by the two world wars, each of which gave a stimulus to research and development as well as bringing significant technological and organizational change to the industry and to individual players in it.

FROM THE LATE NINETEENTH CENTURY TO 1918

Enthusiasm in England for proprietary medicines was noted in the eighteenth century; according to one observer, 'The English are easier than any other nation infatuated by the prospect of universal medicines, nor is there any country in the World where the doctors raise such immense fortunes.'[1] From early in the nineteenth century the manufacturers of universal remedies in pill form, such as Beecham and

168

Holloway, found a large and ready market for their products. Such pills were usually made of a few simple ingredients – aloes, powdered ginger and soap were the constituents of Beecham's pills – although the precise combination was a heavily guarded secret; they were cheap to make, heavily advertised as effective against illnesses ranging from fever to cancer and made fortunes for those who manufactured them.

At the same time advances in medical and scientific knowledge played a part in stimulating the development of a pharmaceutical industry. By later standards its products may seem at best crude, at worst positively dangerous, but they were recognizably pharmaceuticals. As the century wore on, they were also based on a greater understanding of the chemistry of the substances used, both vegetable and mineral. The isolation of morphine from opium in 1806, for example, was followed by the identification of other alkaloids, emetine, strychnine, brucine, quinine, and cinchonine by 1820. Even so, medical practitioners and pharmacists could as yet rarely offer prescriptions which went beyond the relief of pain and of other symptoms of disease.

Expanding demand from a growing and increasingly urban population, with a rising standard of living, helped to fuel the expansion of the industry in the second half of the nineteenth century. While the services of medical practitioners were still too expensive for most working-class pockets, medicines from the pharmacists or chemist and druggist became affordable for more people.

By the 1880s the industry consisted of a number of medium-sized and small businesses. Some were partnerships, some were incorporated but most of them were family-owned or influenced and managed. Their business lay in the importation of raw materials, both vegetable and mineral, from which they extracted and purified the ingredients for drugs. These they then packaged and distributed to wholesalers, to pharmacists, and to medical practitioners both at home and overseas. Some remedies they mixed themselves, supplying them in liquid, powder, or pill form and, more frequently from the 1890s, in tablet form.[2]

Some of them had developed their manufacturing activities out of a retailing business. The firm which became Allen & Hanburys spawned two manufacturing establishments; in 1806 the nine-year-old partnership of Luke Howard and William Allen was amicably dissolved, freeing Howard to build up what became a well-respected chemical manufacturing business, under his own name, in Stratford, East London.[3] In the 1870s Allen & Hanburys itself acquired factory premises in Bethnal Green which allowed the firm to manufacture on a larger scale than its pharmacy in central London had permitted.[4]

Thomas Morson inherited his father's thriving import, wholesale, and retail pharmacy business in Fleet Market and later developed the manufacture of alkaloids, moving to a factory in north London.[5]

Arthur Cox, who had built up a retail pharmacy in Brighton on the strength of a tasteless pill coating which he had invented and patented, handed the shop over to his son in 1871 and established a separate manufacturing business, also in Brighton.[6] Jesse Boot, whose chain of chemists' shops grew from his first base in Nottingham, started a small manufacturing department to supply his shops in 1885; it was, and remained until the end of the century, a small operation, producing some of the then popular proprietary medicines for coughs, colds, and influenza.[7]

Others such as May & Baker[8] and Whiffen & Sons,[9] who both had factories in Battersea, had started as manufacturing chemists and had never been involved in retailing. Relations between these well-established manufacturers were ordered by a spirit of cooperation rather than competition; William Baker of May & Baker told *The Chemist & Druggist* in 1897 that his company had never entered the quinine business, although strongly tempted, because of its 'friendly relations' with Howards. The latter's reputation for quinine was high and it was Howards' most profitable product for most of the nineteenth century.[10]

Competition in the industry was governed by agreements which had increasingly, since the 1880s, covered such products as mercurials, camphor, bismuth, and ether. The 1902 agreement on mercurial preparations was typical of such 'conventions', as they were known, although the parties to it were all British while many of the agreements were international. Five manufacturers established minimum selling prices for mercurial preparations to which they would adhere and agreed to keep a quota market shares of the trade, based on the amounts they had sold in the preceding three and a half years.[11] Cartel agreements setting prices and quotas permeated the heavy chemical industry at this time[12] and became more, rather than, less, common in the fine chemical industry between the wars.[13]

The description of May & Baker's Garden Wharf factory, published in 1889 in *The Chemist & Druggist*, was probably fairly representative of manufacturing operations in the industry at that time.

So we passed straight away into a land of huge retorts and seething furnaces. I was amused with the sight of an iron weight which I could not lift floating buoyantly in a lake of mercury [mercury preparations were then the only known remedy against syphilis and other common venereal diseases]. I choked in the camphor making sheds, which when they periodically catch fire, have simply to be left to burn down and a rare blaze they make. I shuddered as noxious compounds like corrosive sublimate and nitric acid and other *diableries*, to which vitriol is as mother's milk, were dealt with around me by the hogshead and the hundredweight. I was shown a huge tank of pure ether and on holding my hand under the tap was given the sensation of clinging to an iceberg at the North Pole.

In one respect, however, it differed, as the report went on:

Before I left I was made to grasp the difference between sulphonal and . . . phenacetin, a similar white powder which has a direct action on such pains as neuralgia and which presumably is a narcotic. The workmen have sworn by phenacetin ever since it brought relief and sleep to one of them who had burnt his hand with some devil's broth he was stirring.[14]

Phenacetin, a pain-killing drug, was the first pharmaceutical product developed by the German chemical company, Friedrich Bayer & Co., which, in 1888, licensed May & Baker to manufacture and market it in the UK. A year later Bayer introduced the sedative, sulfonal, and again licensed May & Baker to produce it for the British market.[15] The licensing agreement, however, lasted only a few years for Bayer made other arrangements to market its drugs in the UK as its pharmaceutical product portfolio expanded.

The discovery and introduction of these two drugs well illustrates the sharp contrast between the German and the British industries. Phenacetin and sulfonal were the fruit of Bayer's research and development which was, like the company's manufacturing operations and those of its fellow German fine chemical manufacturers, carried out on a scale then unenvisaged in Britain. In the 1880s Bayer employed some 1,000 hands (May & Baker employed about 100 people) as well as nearly 30 chemists in the research department.[16]

Chemistry provided a strong link between dyestuffs and synthetic drugs and Bayer's technical and financial success in the dyestuffs industry underpinned its entry to the pharmaceutical business. In 1896 Bayer established a separate pharmaceutical department which, in the following year, prepared and introduced aspirin. Another German dyestuffs company, Hoechst, had preceded Bayer's entry into the pharmaceutical industry with the introduction of the analgesic, antipyrin. In the 1890s, through collaborating with and supporting the German bacteriologists Emil von Behring and Robert Koch, Hoechst began to manufacture the diphtheria and anti-tetanus serums discovered by Behring.[17]

In Britain from 1895 these biological products were distributed, but not made, by Allen & Hanburys through a connection with the Lister

Institute. They were, however, produced by Evans Sons Lescher & Webb Ltd (later the Evans Medical Company) of Liverpool which had created and cultivated a relationship with medical scientists at Liverpool University. The company also supported the Liverpool Institute of Pathology and, when it closed in 1911, bought its plant and facilities. Evans was unusual in the industry, if not unique at that time, in developing such a connection with a university department, but it did not lead the company into innovation on its own account.[18] Burroughs Wellcome (see below) also manufactured biological products.

Few of the companies, whose origins in the industry have been discussed above, employed at this time more than one or two qualified chemists or pharmacists; and those employed were principally engaged in routine testing of materials and products. Higher standards for the preparation of pharmaceutical ingredients had been set, following the 1858 Medical Act's stipulation that the General Medical Council should produce 'a list of medicines and compounds, and the manner of preparing them, together with true weights and measures by which they are to be prepared and mixed.'[19] The first *British Pharmacopoeia* was published in 1864 and thereafter pharmaceutical and fine chemical manufacturers laid greater emphasis on meeting the standards it set. Similarly in this century the Dangerous Drugs Act of 1922, the Pharmacy and Poisons Act of 1933, and later the Medicines Act of 1968 required higher standards and led to the appointment of more qualified people in the industry.

Cox's, still a very small family business, took on their first qualified chemist in 1904 to work in the dispensing department.[20] In the 1890s Jesse Boot established an analytical laboratory but its small staff were, apart from quality control, concerned mainly with analysing proprietory medicines of competitors in order that Boots should develop new and/or cheaper formulations.[21] Both Whiffens and Morsons established laboratories in the 1880s but neither company went beyond routine sampling and testing.[22]

In the 1890s May & Baker was more preoccupied with a venture into manufacturing cyanide for the gold extraction industry than with a quest for new pharmaceuticals. The venture proved to be a commercial disaster and, in the early years of this century, the company turned its attention again to its old established galenical business and the development of mineral salts. Its scientific expertise remained, however, negligible and it did not at this time employ more than one qualified chemist.[23]

Diversification also appealed to Allen & Hanburys and in the 1890s the company invested heavily in new manufacturing facilities at Ware in Hertfordshire. Although some bulk galenicals – cascara sagrada and liquorice – were produced at Ware, the factory was mainly intended for the milk-based babyfoods and malted products which the company had recently introduced and which had proved very popular in the market. Allen & Hanburys had for some time had a laboratory at its Bethnal Green factory but work undertaken there, as at Howards' factory in east London, was in the 'tradition of gentlemanly puttering in chemistry'.[24] That was far removed from the process of research, discovery, and marketing, already developed in Germany and described in 1913 in terms still largely recognizable today. In the *Chemical News* that year, Carl Duisberg, who had joined Bayer in 1883 as a research chemist and had become, in 1911, chief executive and chairman of what was by 1913 Germany's largest chemical company,[25] wrote:

What an organization, what boundless intelligence is necessary, and what immense energy has to be expended in order to discover a new synthetic remedy and to smooth its path through the obstacles of commerce! First, we need a fully equipped chemical laboratory, then a pharmacological institute with a staff of men trained in medicine and chemistry, an abundance of animals to experiment upon, and finally – the latest development in this field – a chemotherapeutic and bacteriological department, equipped according to the ideas of Paul Ehrlich [see p. 175]: all these must be in close connection with one another. Whatever has been evolved, and after much painstaking effort selected as useful, finds its way into the manufacturing department, there to be elaborated in the most minute details and brought to the highest possible pitch of perfection. Now begins the arduous work of the scientific department! Here the right sponsors must be found, here all prejudices must be brushed aside and an extensive propaganda initiated. Next, a host of clinicians and practitioners must be called into requisition so that what has been evolved in the silent workshop will be conducted on a staunch ship into the wild sea of publicity. And, finally, it is the calculating salesman's turn; he must bring in enough to cover all the expenses of the innumerable experiments that have been made, if the new drug, which has swallowed so much money, is to survive and prosper.[26]

The lack of research facilities and innovation in the British pharmaceutical industry at this time has been ascribed to a number of factors. These include patent legislation less favourable to innovation than that in Germany and the system of technical and scientific education in the UK. Until changes made in the 1880s took effect, there was not, as in Germany, 'a steadily increasing flow of well-trained chemists' coming out of colleges and available for industry.[27] These factors also played a part in the failure of the UK to develop a dyestuffs industry sufficiently technically advanced to compete with that of Germany. Haber's characterization of the industry aptly summarises its state: 'The history of

the British dyestuffs industry is a disappointing story of initial success
[in the 1850s and 1860s] followed by a long but irresistible decline.'[28]
The significance of the dyestuffs industry for the pharmaceutical industry lies not only in the chemical link between them, but also in finance;
dyestuffs were, on the whole, very profitable whereas traditional galenical pharmaceuticals provided only relatively small profit margins.

In the USA also there was no dyestuffs industry to speak of and there
too a traditional pharmaceutical industry, largely based – as in Britain
– on galenical products, had developed by 1880. Over the next two
decades pharmaceutical companies grew rapidly; the application of
scientific, particularly chemical, principles and knowledge to their
operations led to the establishment of analytical laboratories. But, as in
Britain, research on the scale and with the scope of that in Germany did
not exist.[29]

It was, however, from the USA that two pharmaceutical entre-
preneurs came to Britain in 1880 to establish a business that was to play
a major role in the UK industry. Silas Burroughs and Henry Wellcome
had both trained as pharmacists in the USA before they decided to set
up their own business in Britain, principally to exploit the compressed
medicines in tablet form developed successfully in the USA. They
started manufacturing in Britain in the 1880s and in 1889 moved to
Dartford which has been the Wellcome company's main manufacturing
base ever since. They built up a large export trade and, in 1894,
established the Wellcome Physiological Research Laboratories. Two
years later the company, now controlled solely by Henry Wellcome
following Burroughs' death in 1895, set up the Wellcome Chemical
Research Laboratories. The research work and the discoveries made at
the Wellcome Laboratories were significant as also was the role they
played as providers of qualified and experienced research scientists to
other companies, including Boots, Glaxo and May & Baker, in the
industry.

Wellcome himself had a long-standing and keen interest in tropical
diseases which was reflected in the opening in 1902 of the first Wellcome
Tropical Research Laboratory in Khartoum. Wellcome enterprises,
ranging from floating laboratories to overseas branches continued to
mushroom and, although it was not until 1924 that they were consolidated into one private company, the Wellcome Foundation Ltd, a
coordinating body for the separate research establishments was set up
in London in 1913, the Wellcome Bureau of Scientific Research.[30]

The outbreak of war in 1914 abruptly cut off the supplies of drugs and
dyestuffs from Germany. Among these, contributing to the £2m worth
of pharmaceuticals imported in 1913 (£2.4m worth were also exported

that year), were a number of essential medicines. Aspirin was one of the imported drugs and a number of British companies began to manufacture it, including Howards and W. J. Bush, a company which had previously specialized in flavouring essences.[31] Boots also began to manufacture aspirin as well as phenacetin and atropine, after new production facilities had been built and scientifically qualified staff recruited; several of the latter, led by F. H. Carr, came from Wellcome's research laboratories.[32] The shortage of synthetic drugs encouraged other companies to start manufacture; Menley & James, a subsidiary of A. J. White Ltd, which had been marketing and distributing pharmaceutical specialties since 1908, began manufacturing in Camberwell in 1916.[33]

Among the drugs that could no longer be imported from Germany was Salvarsan, the first effective anti-syphilis treatment. It was the result of some years' research work by the bacteriologist, Paul Ehrlich, supported by the fine chemical companies, Cassella and Hoechst. The research had been directed towards finding a 'magic bullet' to attack and destroy the organisms causing the disease. The discovery of the organo-arsenic compounds, salvarsan and neo-salvarsan, was taken up by Hoechst which began commercial production in 1910.[34]

Anticipating that venereal disease would be a problem among the armed forces – in the event it has been estimated that one in five fighting men were infected with syphilis[35] – the British government moved swiftly to secure replacement supplies. The only pharmaceutical company in the UK capable of making the compounds in 1914 was Burroughs, Wellcome & Co, which was licensed by the Board of Trade to make and sell products chemically identical to those of Hoechst under the names of kharsivan and neo-kharsivan. At the same time a second licence was granted to the French company, Société Anonyme des Etablissements Poulenc Frères, for the manufacture of arsenobenzol-billon and novarsenobenzol-billon. The drugs were to be supplied in Britain by May & Baker, who had been agents for Poulenc Frères for some years, and who were also to be helped by Poulenc to start manufacture on their own account. In 1916 May & Baker began to produce the organo-arsenical compounds at a factory in Wandsworth acquired for the purpose.

Manufacture was not without problems:

The preparation of salvarsan [and the British and French arsenical compounds] entailed a multi-stage process starting from aniline or phenol and at each stage, but more seriously at the late stages, side-reactions produced impurities, impossible to prevent and difficult to remove and Ehrlich had therefore established biological tests which all German material had to pass before it was released for use.[36]

In Britain the tests on the organo-arsenic compounds manufactured by Wellcome, Poulenc, and May & Baker were carried out by the Medical Research Committee (later the Medical Research Council), established in 1913. The Committee had looked to Wellcome's Physiological Research Laboratory to staff its research group and recruited three of the team of scientists who had been working on the ergot alkaloids, a project which later led to the discovery of several major new drugs.[37] One of them, Dr Arthur Ewins, was persuaded in 1917 to leave the Medical Research Committee and join May & Baker as Chief Chemist at the Wandsworth factory; his brief was to establish a research and development department for the company.

The First World War then had provided a considerable stimulus to the UK pharmaceutical industry to create a research and development capability.

FROM 1918 TO 1945

In the USA too the war had meant that the pharmaceutical industry was forced into greater self-reliance. This was followed in the years between the wars by the growth of much larger corporations, sometimes by merger, with greater resources to spend on research and development. Merck, now a US company after its severance from its German parent during the war, merged in 1927 with the Philadelphia based pharmaceutical company, Powers–Weightman–Rosengarten. The combined company had sales in 1929 of nearly £3m. By contrast, in the UK Allen & Hanburys' turnover had peaked at over £1m in 1920 but then dropped back; in any case that figure was not attributable solely to pharmaceuticals, including as it did the businesses in infant foods, malted foods, surgical instruments, and other activities, well justifying the description of the company as the 'universal provider'. May & Baker's sales of pharmaceuticals did not reach the £1m mark until 1943. The much smaller company, Arthur H. Cox & Co, specializing in pill manufacture did not achieve sales of £1m until the late 1960s.[38]

In Germany the old-established pharmaceutical companies such as Merck, Schering, and Riedel also grew, partly by the acquisition of other smaller companies. By 1928 Schering and Merck each had some 3,000 employees. At the same time the chemical companies, whose interest in dyestuffs had taken them into the pharmaceutical industry, merged. Bayer, Badische Anilin und Sodafabrik, and Hoechst joined with five other chemical companies in 1925 to form I. G. Farbenindustrie AG; their pharmaceutical operations gave IG Farben a significant place in the industry.[39] The formation of Imperial Chemical

Industries (ICI) in the UK in 1926, a merger of four companies including the British Dyestuffs Corporation, was a response not only to the emergence of IG Farben but also to the creation of large chemical combines in the USA. Most of the resources of ICI, however, until the Second World War, were directed to the heavy chemical sector and pharmaceuticals were largely ignored by the company.[40]

For the pharmaceutical companies in Britain whose origins and business before 1914 has been explored, demand for the old traditional products continued to be strong. The consumer's appetite for proprietary medicines was reflected in the growth of sales and profits of companies such as Beecham which had introduced Beecham's Powders in 1926. Although the company itself employed (from 1924) only one analytical chemist, its profits enabled it to fund, from 1937, the Beecham Laboratory at the Royal Northern Hospital in London. The company's entry into the pharmaceutical industry proper, however, and the establishment of its own research and development department, did not take place until during the Second World War.[41] Side by side, however, with the production of proprietary products there was at this time a growing research and development capacity and an increasing number of new drugs being introduced on the market.

One of the first of these was insulin, a hormonal treatment for diabetes successfully developed and introduced in Canada in 1922. The commercial production of insulin in Britain was undertaken by four companies, by agreement with the Medical Research Council which had been given the British rights to the patents. The four companies were Boots, Wellcome, British Drug Houses, and Allen & Hanburys. The two last established a partnership in 1923 with the manufacture being undertaken by British Drug Houses (BDH), and analytical work and packing by Allen & Hanburys. BDH, created by the merger of several wholesale drug houses in 1908, had set up manufacturing facilities and inaugurated research and development, with the acquisition of F. H. Carr and his team of research chemists (originally from Wellcome) when they left Boots in 1918.[42]

After Carr and his assistants left Boots the company had only four research chemists until 1927 when a new head of the research laboratory was recruited. Dr F. L. Pyman from Manchester University, formerly with Wellcome's Research Laboratory, brought five research chemists with him to Boots. The company was then, and until 1933, owned by the American United Drug Company. However, after its return to English ownership, the interests of Jesse Boot's son, the second Lord Trent, whose autocratic rule of the company lasted from 1933 until 1954, lay with the retailing side. Manufacturing and research and development therefore remained the 'Cinderella of the business'.[43]

For Wellcome, its historian has written, the interwar years were 'a period of some stagnation'. The company's reputation, however, remained high and it was the first to manufacture insulin in the UK. In the Development Laboratories the cardiac glycoside, digitoxin, was isolated from the leaves of *digitalis lanata*[44] and there were some innovations in tropical medicines. Probably the two most significant developments in the British pharmaceutical industry during the interwar years were, first, the results achieved by the newly established research department at May & Baker and, secondly, the arrival in the industry of a newcomer in the shape of Glaxo.

Under the leadership of Dr Arthur Ewins (see page 176) May & Baker's research staff had expanded in the years immediately after the war. By 1927 there were four qualified chemists and two pharmacists at the Wandsworth factory and laboratory as well as six assistants, some of whom were of graduate ability and working for degrees part time. The company had benefited from its association with Poulenc Frères, whose research laboratory had been established in 1903 and where the French chemist Ernest Fourneau had worked until 1911, when he became head of the chemotherapeutic laboratory at the Pasteur Institute. May & Baker's Wandsworth factory started to manufacture Poulenc specialties, which included anaesthetics and vaccines as well as the arsenical compounds made during the war. In 1925 the factory also started to manufacture, under licence from the American Rockefeller Institute, the drug tryparsamide, developed by the Institute to combat sleeping sickness.

The death of the major family shareholders in May & Baker soon after the end of the First World War led to an agreement in 1927 for Poulenc Frères to buy May & Baker (Poulenc already had a shareholding in the company). However, in 1928 Poulenc Frères itself merged with the Société Chimique des Usines du Rhône and the latter completed the purchase of May & Baker. The decision to build a new factory at Dagenham was, therefore, taken by Rhône-Poulenc in 1932. Constructed to French plans and with French technical advice, the factory was ready for May & Baker to move into in April 1934.

In 1935 Gerhard Domagk, a research director at I. G. Farben, used the azo dye, prontosil, whose therapeutic effect he had been exploring, to save the life of his daughter who was suffering from septicaemia. A year later work started in May & Baker's research department on the sulphonamide group of compounds and, late in 1937, compound number 693 – M & B 693 – was synthesized. Tests quickly showed it to be effective against bacterial pneumonia, for which previously there had been no cure, and it was used extensively in the years immediately before and during the war. The research department continued to work on the sulphonamide drugs, developing a number of other compounds in the group although none with the impact of M & B 693.[45] May & Baker's reputation within the British pharmaceutical industry and beyond was considerably enhanced by the discovery of M & B 693. It has never been easy to measure innovation and research and development performance; patenting activity provides one indicator and between 1936 and 1941 May & Baker took out forty patents as against Burroughs Wellcome's six, seven from BDH and Boots and Glaxo (see below) taking out twelve and thirteen respectively.[46]

It was not only, however, in the fields of new biological products and new synthetic drugs that discoveries were made in the interwar years. Since the 1870s research had been going on into what were at first called 'accessory food factors' and later became known as vitamins.[47] The work on vitamins attracted the attention of the Glaxo department of J. E. Nathan & Company. The Nathan company, owned by a family of merchants and traders in New Zealand, had started the manufacture of dried milk in the early years of this century and found, by trial and error, that the best market for it was babyfood. Demand for Glaxo babyfood, introduced in 1908, increased during the First World War but the poor quality of some of the dried milk led Alec Nathan, the brother most concerned with that part of the business, to employ Harry Jephcott, a chemist and pharmacist by profession, to deal with the problem.[48]

With Alfred Bacharach, recruited from Wellcome, and two other qualified staff, Jephcott established a laboratory and quality control procedures for Glaxo babyfood. He then turned their attention to research work being done in nutritional science, much of it in the USA. During a visit to the USA in 1923 Jephcott secured a licence to use the process developed by Dr Theodore Drucker of Columbia University for the extraction of vitamin D. In the following year the Glaxo department of Nathans manufactured and introduced vitamin D, its first pharmaceutical product. Five years later Glaxo took a licence, again from the USA, for an improved process (the Steenbock process) for manufacturing vitamin D by irradiating ergosterol.

Through the 1930s Glaxo added other vitamin products to its small range of pharmaceuticals and sold them overseas as well as at home. This led, as it had done with other pharmaceutical companies such as Allen & Hanburys and May & Baker, to the establishment of overseas subsidiaries, mainly in the countries of the British Empire, Australia,

Canada, India, and South Africa. For the Glaxo department further expansion was constrained by its small research staff and the poor financial results of its parent company. Nor were the Nathan brothers, except Alec, wholeheartedly committed to pharmaceutical manufacture, although it offered larger profit margins than other diversifications the company had made into retailing in the UK and in New Zealand. Jephcott therefore looked (in the main to the USA but also to Norway) for products for which Glaxo would be able to secure a licence to manufacture. His research staff concentrated on process development, a training that was to stand them in good stead during and after the Second World War.

Glaxo's spending on long-term research in the late 1930s averaged about £5,000 a year, spread among a number of projects including an attempt to synthesize vitamin A; that amount was clearly considered by those concerned to be too little but more was not, apparently, available. After Glaxo was incorporated as a private company in 1935, it established close relations with several university chemistry departments and, by the end of the decade, with a new, purpose-built factory and laboratories at Greenford, it had established itself in the industry.

Despite the progress that the industry as a whole had made during the interwar years, the outbreak of war in 1939 once again cut off supplies of drugs hitherto imported from Germany. The most effective anti-malarial drug, atebrin, was a German product and at the Government's instigation Boots, ICI, and May & Baker cooperated in developing anti-malarials, especially mepacrine. At Greenford Glaxo analysed, researched, developed, and produced substitutes for German radiographic media and anaesthetics.

The war also led to the formation of a cooperative research organization, the Therapeutic Research Corporation (TRC), which was established in 1941. The brainchild of Burroughs Wellcome's chairman, T. R. G. Bennett, TRC's members initially were Boots, BDH, Burroughs Wellcome, Glaxo, and May & Baker. In 1942, ICI set up a pharmaceuticals division which also became a member of the TRC. Collaboration, however, was not easy to achieve, TRC's members found, given the well-established habits of competition, secrecy, and suspicion as far as research and new products were concerned, but the TRC did play an important role in the development of penicillin production in Britain during the war.[49]

THE THERAPEUTIC REVOLUTION: FROM 1945 TO THE 1960s

The research and development initiative in the international pharmaceutical industry clearly passed to the USA during the war. Penicillin production by deep fermentation rather than the surface culture method used in Britain was developed by Merck and Squibb as well as by Pfizer, a newcomer to the industry. Merck also introduced strepto-mycin, effective against tuberculosis and other diseases and went on to beat Glaxo, narrowly, in identifying vitamin B_{12}, the anti-pernicious anaemia factor. Parke Davis discovered the first broad-spectrum anti-biotic, chloramphenicol, in 1947 and others, including tetracycline in 1953, discovered by Pfizer and Cyanamid, soon followed. Some 60% of new drugs discoveries between 1941 and 1963 originated in the USA, nearly 8% in Switzerland, nearly 6% in Germany and just under 5% in the UK.[50] This overwhelming US dominance fell in the 1970s and between 1970 and 1983 the US industry accounted for some 40% of new introductions.[51] In Germany I. G. Farben was broken up after the war and Bayer, Badische, and Hoechst reemerged as separate com-panies; in Switzerland the companies that eventually became CIBA–Geigy and Hoffman–La Roche were the major players.

In the years immediately after 1945 UK pharmaceutical companies, anxious to develop and expand their activities, found themselves inhi-bited from doing so by the state of the economy, the wartime controls that remained in place, and government attitudes and policies. Short-ages of everything from sterling to construction materials limited their ability to repair war damage and build new facilities in the short term; their choices of new factory locations and sources of raw materials were also restricted. By the end of the war Glaxo was the largest UK supplier of penicillin and the company moved swiftly to secure, by agreements with Merck and Squibb, access to the US technology of deep fermen-tation penicillin. The location of Glaxo's new penicillin factory at Barnard Castle, however, was the government's, rather than the com-pany's, choice and added to production costs. The government was also able to exert a downward pressure on penicillin prices although by 1950 that was no longer necessary as increased production worldwide contri-buted to dramatic falls in all penicillin product prices. In the 1950s vaccine prices were kept low by the government's setting prices and the industry was pressed to find supplies of raw materials, for example for cortisone drugs, in the sterling rather than the dollar area.[52]

The introduction of the National Health Service in 1948 increased the demand for medicines and at the same time it gave the government a close and continuing interest in the prices that pharmaceutical companies were charging. Through the 1950s and the 1960s the indus-try lived with constant scrutiny, from the investigations of the Guille-baud Committee into the cost of the NHS in 1956, through those of the Hinchcliffe Committee in 1959, to the Sainsbury Committee on the relationship between the industry and the NHS in 1967. The public concern aroused by the inquiries of the Kefauver Committee in the USA in 1961 also had repercussions in the UK.

In the industry views on the prospects for the expansion of research and development varied. May & Baker started work on a new research institute in 1954 and it was completed in 1960; by then it housed some 350 full-time research workers. The company benefited from a new agreement signed after the war with its parent, Rhône–Poulenc, for technology access and licensing and was able to introduce a number of new products in the 1950s.[53] Wellcome emerged from its pre-war stagnation about 1950 and acquired new research and development facilities at Beckenham. Beecham expanded its laboratory significantly in the 1950s, started work on penicillin in 1954, and in 1959 launched the first of the new semi-synthetic penicillins on the market.[54]

At Glaxo the prevailing view was more pessimistic: Jephcott's conviction that only by 'increased efficiency gained with little or no capital expenditure . . . industry can best aid the national economic problem and ward off inflationary pressure' underpinned his approach to expenditure on research and development. At Glaxo the emphasis remained on process improvement and productivity enhancement at the expense of long-term speculative research. Even so Glaxo's annual research expenditure was, the company told the Guillebaud Committee in 1952, between £450,000 and £500,000, a figure much the same as those of ICI and Wellcome, although the latter only spent some 60% of the total in the UK. Until the 1970s Glaxo depended heavily on, and paid not insubstantial sums for, licences from US companies to manufacture new products.

It was the US companies that Glaxo chose to measure itself against in the 1950s; the comparison revealed that whatever yardstick was used, Glaxo was much smaller than the eight US corporations. They employed more capital, had larger turnovers and profits, enjoyed higher profit margins and allocated greater proportions of the profits to research and development.[55] An increasing number of them also, along with German and Swiss companies, were seeking to establish subsidiaries in the UK, either directly or by acquisition of the smaller UK companies. In the two decades after the war there was considerable restructuring in the UK industry and many of the old-established companies, whose origins and development have been discussed, disappeared. They were not all acquired by foreign companies; Fisons bought Whiffen in 1947 and tried, but failed, to buy BDH. Howards became part of Laporte Industries Ltd in 1961. Cox's, which had surprisingly survived as a family-owned company, remained independent until 1984 when it was bought by Hoechst.

Fear of their vulnerability to US predators led to the merger in 1958 of Glaxo and Allen & Hanburys. Two years later the unwelcome approaches of a UK predator, Fisons, to the Evans Medical Company led to the acquisition of Evans by the Glaxo group. As Evans' chairman noted regretfully, 'the trend towards larger and ever larger units . . . cannot be avoided and must, therefore, be accepted'.[56]

CONCLUSION

Glaxo followed the acquisitions discussed above with those of the Edinburgh Pharmaceutical Industries in 1962, the British Drug Houses Group in 1967, and Farleys Infant Food in 1968. Four years later, despite the size of the Group, it found itself the unwelcome target of a takeover bid from Beecham. The bid, and the proposed alternative defensive alliance that Glaxo had swiftly made with Boots, were referred to the Monopolies Commission which rejected both as not in the best interests of the industry. The Commission took the view that the size and market power of either combination would reduce, rather than increase, innovation. Some empirical research since then has confirmed the conclusion that size may not inevitably correlate with best research and development performance.[57]

From the mid-1960s Glaxo began to direct resources to basic long-term research and, at the same time, started to review its international operations and relationships. The latter led to a decision in 1972 to develop its operations and presence in the Japanese market. It also led to the cancellation of Glaxo's long-term agreements with the US company, Schering-Plough, and, in 1978, the acquisition of Meyer Laboratories Inc. in Florida and entry to the US market. These moves, combined with a steady flow of introductions of new products in the 1970s and 1980s resulting from the company's research programme, were followed by a period of remarkable growth for Glaxo.[58] In the 1980s the company rose from ranking as the world's twentieth largest company (in 1981) to become the second largest, close on the heels of Merck.

Over the last two decades research and development costs have spiralled. At the same time governments have pressed for reductions in drug prices because of the increasing costs of healthcare in the USA and in Europe where the population structure includes a larger proportion of older people. The rate of growth enjoyed by the industry – nearly 10% a year between 1963 and 1972 – has slowed down, as has the rate of discovery; ninety-three new medicines were launched in 1961, forty-eight in 1980. In the mid-1980s a new period of international restructuring began with more than ten mergers, including that of SmithKline Beckman with Beecham in 1989, taking place and the debate about the relationship between size and research and development performance has resurfaced.[59]

NOTES

This account of research and development in the UK pharmaceutical industry is built on two papers given by the author. The first, covering the interwar years, was presented at the Annual Conference of the Association of Business Historians at Leeds University, 9–10 July 1993, and the second, on the period after the Second World War, at the LSE, Business History Unit Symposium, supported by the Wellcome Trust, on 19 November 1993.

1 Mrs Montagu, quoted in W. A. Campbell, *The Chemical Industry* (Harlow, 1971) p. 116.

2 Machinery to compress drug constituents into tablets was developed in Germany and in the USA in the 1880s and 1890s. The US methods were brought to Britain by Burroughs Wellcome & Co. which registered the word 'Tabloid' as its trademark in 1884. See G. Macdonald, *In Pursuit of Excellence. Wellcome 1880–1980* (Wellcome Foundation, London, 1980).

3 G. Tweedale, *At the Sign of the Plough. Allen & Hanburys and the British Pharmaceutical Industry 1715–1990* (Stanford in the Vale, 1990) pp. 33–5. See also P. J. T. Morris and C. A. Russell, ed. J. Graham Smith, *Archives of the British Chemical Industry 1750–1914* (British Society for the History of Science, Stanford in the Vale, 1988), pp. 103–4.

4 Tweedale, *Allen & Hanburys*, pp. 72–3.

5 J. Liebenau, *Morson, Thomas*, in D. Jeremy, ed., *Dictionary of Business Biography*, IV (London, 1985), pp. 346–7.

6 J. A. Slinn, *Pills and Pharmaceuticals. A. H. Cox Co Ltd 1839–1989* (A. H. Cox & Co. Ltd., 1989).

7 S. Chapman, *Jesse Boote of Boots the Chemists* (London, 1974), pp. 61–2.

8 J. A. Slinn, *A History of May & Baker 1834–1984* (Cambridge, 1984).

9 J. Liebenau, *Whiffen, Thomas*, in D. Jeremy, ed., *Dictionary of Business Biography*, V (London, 1986), pp. 763–5.

10 Quoted in Slinn, *May & Baker*. For Howards and quinine, see Morris and Russell, *Archives of the British Chemical Industry*, p. 103.

11 GLC Archives, Whiffen Archives. B/WHF/25.

12 See W. J. Reader, *Imperial Chemical Industries: A History*, I (Oxford, 1970).

13 See L. F. Haber, *The Chemical Industry 1900–1930* (Oxford, 1971), p. 272.

14 *The Chemist & Druggist*, 4 May 1889, p. 613.

15 For Bayer, see L. F. Haber, *The Chemical Industry during the Nineteenth Century* (Oxford, 1958), pp. 134–5. Slinn, *May & Baker*.

16 For Tyrer's visit see Slinn, *May & Baker*. For Bayer see J. Liebenau, 'Industrial Research & Development in Pharmaceutical Firms in the Early Twentieth Century', *Business History*, 26, 3 (November 1984), pp. 327–46. Also Haber, *Chemical Industry during the Nineteenth Century*, pp. 132–3.

17 Haber, *Chemical Industry during the Nineteenth Century*, pp. 132–3.

18 Liebenau, 'Industrial Research & Development'.

19 L. G. Matthews, *History of Pharmacy in Britain* (London, 1962), pp. 67–88.

20 Slinn, *Pills and Pharmaceuticals*.

21 Chapman, *Boots the Chemists*.

22 Liebenau, *Dictionary of Business Biography*, IV and V: Entries on Morson and Whiffen.

23 Slinn, *May & Baker*.

24 For Allen & Hanburys, see Tweedale, *Allen & Hanburys*; quotation from Liebenau, 'Industrial Research & Development'.

25 For Duisberg, see Haber, *Chemical Industry in the Nineteenth Century*, pp. 187–8 and Haber, *Chemical Industry 1900–1930*, p. 128.

26 *Chemical News*, 23 May 1913, pp. 246–7. Quoted in Liebenau, 'Industrial Research & Development'.

27 Haber, *Chemical Industry during the Nineteenth Century*, p. 71.

28 *Ibid.*, p. 162.

29 Liebenau, 'Industrial Research & Development', and *Medical Science and Medical Industry* (London, 1987).

30 Macdonald, *Wellcome 1880–1980*.

31 Haber, *Chemical Industry 1900–1930*, p. 150. For Howards see Morris and Russell, *Archives of the British Chemical Industry*, p. 103.

32 Chapman, *Boots the Chemists*, pp. 96–7. Following a dispute with Boot, Carr left the company in 1918 and, taking with him some of his team, went to British Drug Houses, p. 141.

33 Morris and Russell, *Archives of the British Chemical Industry*, p. 207.

34 Haber, *Chemical Industry 1900–1930*, pp. 131–2.

35 A. J. P. Taylor, *English History 1914–45* (Oxford, 1965), p. 121. For salvarsan, see also M. Robson, 'The British Pharmaceutical Industry and the First World War', in J. Liebenau, ed., *The Challenge of New Technology: Innovation in British Business since 1850* (Aldershot, 1988), pp. 83–105.

36 H. J. Barber, *Historical Aspects of Chemotherapy* (May & Baker, 1978) p. 12.

37 Macdonald, *Wellcome 1880–1980*, p. 73.

38 For Merck, see *Merck Sharp & Dohme. A Brief History* (MSD, 1992). For Allen & Hanburys see Tweedale, and for May & Baker and Cox's see Slinn.

39 Haber, *Chemical Industry 1900–30*, pp. 284–9.

40 W. J. Reader, *Imperial Chemical Industries A History*, II (Oxford, 1975).

41 M. Robson, 'The Pharmaceutical Industry' (PhD thesis, London University, 1989), I, p. 38. See also H. G. Lazell, *From Pills to Penicillin. The Beecham Story* (London, 1975), and T. A. B. Corley, *The Beecham Group in the World's Pharmaceutical Industry 1914–1970*, paper at the Association of Business Historians' conference, Leeds, July 1993, to be published in *Business History*.

42 For insulin see Tweedale, *Allen & Hanburys*, pp. 127–30. For Carr's departure, see Chapman, *Boots the Chemists*, p. 141.

43 Chapman, *Boots the Chemist*, p. 193.

44 Macdonald, *Wellcome 1880–1980*, pp. 29–30, 74–5.

45 Slinn, *May & Baker*, pp. 122–6.

46 Robson, 'The Pharmaceutical Industry', p. 16.

47 For a summary of this research see R. T. P. Davenport-Hines and Judy Slinn, *Glaxo: A History to 1962* (Cambridge, 1992), pp. 68–71.

48 For this and the following account of Glaxo's entry into the pharmaceutical industry, see *ibid.*

49 For penicillin's discovery and development in the UK, see *ibid.*, ch. 6 and sources quoted p. 385. For the TRC's role see J. Liebenau, 'The British Success with Penicillin', *Social Studies of Science*, 17 (1987), pp. 69–86.

50 W. D. Reekie, *The Economics of the Pharmaceutical Industry* (London, 1975), p. 24.

51 See R. Ballance, J. Pogany, and H. Forstner, *The World's Pharmaceutical Industries* (Newent, 1992), p. 88. The table shows Switzerland in second place with 12.9%, Germany and the UK with 10% each and Sweden, Italy, and Japan assuming a greater role.

52 See Davenport-Hines and Slinn, *Glaxo*, pp. 186–9.

53 Slinn, *May & Baker*, ch. 8.

54 Macdonald, *Wellcome 1880–1980*, pp. 75–7. For Beechams see Corley's paper.

55 Davenport-Hines and Slinn, *Glaxo*, pp. 167–9.

56 Quoted in *ibid.*, p. 173.

57 See Reekie, *Economics of the Pharmaceutical Industry*, pp. 114–16.

58 See Sir Paul Girolami, *The Development of Glaxo* (Glaxo Holdings, 1990). A project led by Dr Edgar Jones looking at the last thirty years of Glaxo's activities is currently underway at the Business History Unit, LSE.

59 See Ballance, Pogany, and Forstner, *The World's Pharmaceutical Industries*, ch. 4 and pp. 183–6.

TEN

AIDS, DRUGS, AND HISTORY

VIRGINIA BERRIDGE

AIDS, in its early years in particular was a disease surrounded by history. Historians actively sought to bring the 'lesson of history' into the public debates. Even more surprisingly, policy makers were often prepared to listen. This essay will examine the various stages of the historical consciousness around AIDS (from the initial stage of 'epidemic disease' to the current period of normalization), will analyse of what the historical input has consisted, and will analyse, too, why history was initially so important. This historical consciousness has not, so far as AIDS is concerned, been applied to drug policy. Drugs have in the past, been an historically conscious area of health policy. But the impact of AIDS on drug policy has tended, in contrast, to be viewed ahistorically, as if all developments were totally new. Why this has been the case gives some insights into the uses of history as a policy-relevant science. This essay will also argue that history has a role to play in the analysis of post-AIDS drug policy – not least in drawing out some distinct themes and continuities with the pre-AIDS situation.

AIDS AND HISTORY: THE EARLY YEARS

The initial historical input into AIDS was marked. In the late twentieth century, laboratory and clinical science appeared to have conquered infectious, epidemic disease. According to the McKeown thesis (which stressed the role of nutrition rather than medical technology in conquering disease), medical discoveries and therapies may not have caused the decline in mortality of the nineteenth century, but they did have a significant impact in the twentieth.[1] Most text books of medical history referred to the shift from infectious to chronic disease – cancer, heart disease – as the major causes of mortality in the twentieth century. There seemed little likelihood that this pattern would change. But suddenly it did. In the early 1980s, a range of societies were confronted

with a major new infectious disease – AIDS – which seemed likely to
develop into a heterosexual epidemic. In Africa, it already was a
heterosexual epidemic. There were no preexisting networks of information, standard procedures, established areas of expertise. The links
the disease had with 'deviant minorities' – blacks, gays, drug users –
seemed likely to call forth hostile social reactions. AIDS was an open
policy area at that stage and a wide range of policy input was possible.
As such, history was seen as having a role to play. Reference to the story
of past epidemics might give some notion of how societies had coped,
what strategies to avoid – even what the end of this particular epidemic
story might be.

The historical input in those early AIDS years concentrated in three
distinct areas. It looked to 'historical parallels' in terms of how past
societies had coped with epidemic disease – for example the cholera
epidemics in England or Germany in the nineteenth century, the Black
Death in fourteenth-century Europe, or plague in Renaissance Florence.[2] Parallels were drawn with the social dislocation likely to be
caused by a major epidemic; with potential population change; or the
possibility of overt hostility to deviant minorities. A second form of
historical input looked specifically at the historical record in the area of
sexually transmitted disease – for although AIDS was an infectious
disease, it was also a sexually transmitted one. Historians drew attention to the historical relationship between such diseases and stigmatized
minorities – prostitutes, blacks. Others used that history to draw a
particular contemporary lesson – the need for a non-punitive approach
to HIV-positive people, and an approach which was based on voluntarism.[3] Of particular importance in the British context was the example
of the nineteenth-century Contagious Diseases Acts, which had
attempted – and failed – to police the transmission of sexually transmitted diseases through enforcement of the 'double standard' of sexual
morality (prostitutes, but not their customers, were medically examined and quarantined). Thereafter – and after further developments
during the First World War – British policy in this area had been
voluntaristic and confidential.[4]

The example of the Contagious Diseases Acts indicates a third form
of historical input – the history of public health initiatives, and in
particular historical illustrations of the complex conflicts in the health
field between the public good and individual liberty. Discussion of
examples such as the struggles over compulsory vaccination in the
nineteenth century seemed appropriate when talk of quarantine and
the isolation of AIDS sufferers was in the air and public fear was at its
height.[5] The range of historical material brought to bear was great.

One article can stand as an example. In December 1986, the historian Roy Porter wrote an editorial in the *British Medical Journal*. Headed 'History Says No to the Policeman's Response to AIDS', it argued strongly, using the historical precedent of the Contagious Diseases Acts, against adding AIDS to the list of notifiable diseases.[6]

Historical precedent says 'no'. For unlike casually contagious diseases, sexually transmitted diseases constitute a special case in which the direct methods of the law have been tried, found wanting, and abandoned . . . Desperate diseases may require desperate remedies. Faced with the enormity of the suffering AIDS will inflict, humanity demands that we at least consider draconian measures such as compulsory screening for suspected virus carriers and further stops to protect others.
Experience suggests, however, that this would be unwise.

This editorial, unlike many based on historical perspectives, attracted considerable interest.[7] For arguments such as these were not, at that stage, simply academic. In the British context, at least, the historical input does appear to have had a policy impact. The public health specialty in Britain has traditionally been an historically conscious one. Both Sir Donald Acheson, the government Chief Medical Officer and the British Medical Association used the historical record in the area of sexually transmitted disease as an argument for voluntarism in evidence to the House of Commons Social Services Committee in 1987.[8] Such considerations also entered into the debates in 1985 around whether or not AIDS should be made a notifiable disease.[9]

THE 'NORMALIZATION' OF HISTORY

Why was history so prominent in the early stages of AIDS policy development? It has already been suggested that AIDS was an open policy area. Established lines of proceeding were yet to be established. As such, the 'lesson of history' was more eagerly invited than is normally the case. And for various reasons, discussed elsewhere, historians themselves were more willing than they had previously been to play an active policy-relevant role.[10] Whether this form of input was indeed an appropriate use for history is a matter for debate. Certainly most historians would have argued that historical input was important. But some saw that input to be more appropriately the opening up of discussion around the nature of the issues involved rather than using the historical record to point a very direct 'lesson'. Some historians saw the latter as a misuse of history, negating the whole nature of the subject.

In the years succeeding this initial phase of historical consciousness, the type of input has changed. What has happened since is a change in the form of historical input. AIDS, in the last two years, has moved from an 'epidemic' to a 'normal' or chronic model of disease. The threat of an immediate heterosexual epidemic has receded. The disease has become normalized and institutionalized. Paid professional workers have replaced the early volunteers; a model of 'chronic disease', with long-term medication with AZT has replaced the early concepts of rapidly terminal illness.[11] As a result the 'epidemic history' of the early years no longer has much of a role to play. 'Historical parallels' have, so it is argued, outlived their usefulness now the immediate emergency has passed. The period of immediate historical consciousness has gone. But some historians have begun to delineate a new role for themselves in the study of AIDS, one which has implications, through AIDS, for the study of health policy in general. That role is not confined to 'historical perspective' or to 'the lesson of history'. It focuses instead on the role historians and historical methods can play in the analysis of the contemporary AIDS story.[12] Of what does this historical input currently consist? As we grow more reflective and less crisis-ridden about the disease, the longer-term perspective has come into play and questions present themselves. For example, how much change has AIDS brought about and how much was inherent in the preexisting policies and situation? How much is continuity and how much change? To answer those types of questions, we need pre-histories of the areas with which AIDS has intersected. But there is also another dimension to contemporary history. Historians can become policy scientists, analysing not just events in the distant past, but also in the very recent past, 'contemporary history' indeed. This type of investigation has begun in several countries and involves historians and other disciplines. In the US a history of Centers for Disease Control's response to AIDS is being written; in the UK, there is a study of the development of AIDS policies overall.[13] The development of AIDS policies is being looked at in cross-national perspective.[14] 'Pre-history' studies have looked, for example, at the problems of pharmaceutical research in wartime and drawn parallels with AIDS; or at hepatitis B as, in some respects, a precursor of AIDS.[15] The function of such contemporary history can vary according to the practitioner and the location. Historians study the past in many cases simply because it happened; there is no reason why that historical consciousness cannot apply to the analysis of recent events as much as to those long distant in time although the balance of available data will be different. The second function is what has been called 'slow journalism', learning the inside story of what really happened. And finally, there is the practical policy-relevant function – that contemporary history offers not a direct lesson, but a methodology to analyse and evaluate policy which policy makers can use. In Britain, this latter function remains problematic, at least from the perspective of departmental research funders.

DRUGS: HISTORY AND THE 1960s

Drugs, too, are part of the AIDS story. How has the period of historical consciousness affected the area of drugs and drug policy under the impact of AIDS? The answer is not a lot. Drugs has been an area where in the past there has been a clear historical input into policy making. In the 1960s and 1970s, at another time of policy flux, the historical record was brought into play. The focus was American drug policy. Attempts to liberalize American drug policy and to introduce methadone maintenance, outpatient treatment, and a role for doctors, turned to the contrast between British and American experience for justification. How this came about needs a brief explanation. The United States in the 1920s adopted a penal system of narcotic control. Legal decisions under the 1914 Harrison Narcotics Act established that maintenance prescribing was not legitimate. Addicts were thrown on the resources of the black market operated by the criminal underworld and doctors who prescribed to them were liable to end up in prison. Not until the 1950s and 60s were moves made to substitute disease views of addiction and medical treatment for criminal prosecution. Marie Nyswander's *The Drug Addict as Patient* (1956) and the report of the joint committee of the American Bar Association and the American Medical Association (1958) argued for a medical approach. The 'British System' which offered the possibility of medical maintenance prescribing was seen as a shining example of the possibilities of medical control. The Rolleston Report of 1926, which had confirmed the legitimacy of such prescribing options was, it was argued, the cause of Britain's small addict population.[16] Reformers like Troy Duster and Edwin Schur looked to the British system as an ideal, and cited the history of its origins in contrast to the 'wrong turning' taken by the United States.[17] The political visibility of history was such that, at one stage, two American funding agencies, the Drug Abuse Council and the National Institute on Drug Abuse, were supporting major studies of the history of British drug policy. There was interest in the short-lived outpatient prescribing clinics established in some American cities in the 1920s; the implications for American drug policy in the 1960s and 70s were clear.[18]

As a result, the history of British drug policy in the 1920s and after emerged as a powerful rhetorical symbol in the minds of policy reformers. Rolleston and the 1920s provided the type of 'lesson of history' for drug policy in the 1960s which the Contagious Diseases Acts provided for AIDS in the 1980s. Forces which sought to redefine drugs as a problem for medical treatment and control rather than for the criminal justice system used Rolleston as an historical exemplar. The story of the 1920s in Britain demonstrated, so it was argued, how Britain had drawn back at the brink of a penal approach. It had, instead, adopted a medical system and had been rewarded by forty years of low addict numbers and minimal criminal involvement. Rolleston became the 'lesson of history' for US drug policy. But history, as this essay has argued, is more than a question of lessons. Historical knowledge proceeds by the statement and testing of hypotheses. And, in the case of drugs, sustained historical research has tended to cast some doubt on the traditional interpretations. In the US, for example, prohibition of drugs under the Harrison Act was not the only important factor. David Courtwright's researches have shown that drug use had been associated with crime and the black market since the end of the nineteenth century.[19] And, in Britain, was the 'British system' that medical; and was it indeed the cause of Britain's small number of addicts? British research has stressed that the medical system operated within an overall structure of Home Office and international control.[20] In essence it was the result and not the cause of the small addict numbers, what David Downes has called 'a system of masterly inactivity in face of a non-existent problem'.[21] Doctors wanted a medical prescribing system so they could maintain their relationship with their middle-class clientele. But this interplay of historical interpretation – the real 'lesson of history' – has had a relatively small impact in a policy sense. The symbolic importance of the 1920s events has outweighed it. In Britain, for example, when debate again began around drug policy in the late 1970s, the traditional interpretations of Rolleston were revived.[22] History, so it seemed, could only provide one message and not an indication of the complexities of policy development.

AIDS AND DRUGS: THE ABSENCE OF HISTORY?

The impact of AIDS on drug policy has not brought forth the historical debates which marked the earlier period of policy flux. The emphasis has tended to be on the essential newness of the impact of AIDS on mechanisms of drug control. A recent paper on British AIDS policies sees the area of drug policy as the one example of how previous aims have been overthrown.[23] Other commentators have stressed how drugs have, for the first time, in the British context, come 'in from the cold' and have been allied to the mainstream concerns of public health.[24]

HIV has simplified the debate and we now see the emergence of what I will call the public health paradigm. Rather than seeing drug use as a metaphorical disease, there is now a real medical problem associated with injecting drugs. All can agree that this is a major public health problem for people who inject drugs, their sexual partners, and their children.

Why this has been so is debatable. AIDS, as a new and open policy area, invited a wide range of initial historical input. AIDS has also served to throw drug policy into a state of flux – or at least to heighten and intensify the tensions which already existed. Yet historical input has been mostly absent. This essay will argue that there are distinct continuities in policy – but that policy objectives in this instance would not have been served by an emphasis on historical perspective.

Current British policy exemplifies some distinct continuities with previous developments; AIDS has served to highlight aspects which have a long history. At a time of policy flux, there has been a natural tendency to stress the newness of policy objectives and means of carrying them out. The apparent newness of objectives in the drugs area has in fact been one means of ensuring their acceptability. But there are also continuities and historical comparisons to be drawn. This essay will focus on four: the role of normalization and harm-minimization; the recurrence of drugs as a 'public health' question; comparisons between the 'epidemic' of the 1960s and that of the 1980s and finally the role of the medical and associated professions in drug policy. Normalization and harm-minimization have been singled out as the keys to post-AIDS British drug policy. The assertion that the danger of the spread of AIDS from drug users into the general population is a greater threat to the nation's health than the dangers of drug misuse itself has been the foundation of the new developments. At least 100 needle exchanges offering new for used syringes provide a tangible expression of new developments. These needle exchanges have provided an embryo national system paralleling and extending that of the clinics.[25] Drug services have come out of the ghetto and the process of integration into the normal range of services has been intensified. Services have been encouraged to become oriented towards clients' needs, including the prescribing of opiates, rather than testing motivation with long waiting lists and abstinence-oriented treatment philosophies.

But are these objectives in essence all that new? The immediate history of drug policy prior to AIDS shows that these were policy objectives in the health sphere even prior to AIDS, as for example in the 1984 ACMD Report on *Prevention*;[26] what AIDS has done is to give them political legitimacy and acceptability. Looked at from a longer-term perspective, it is the post-Brain decade of the late 60s to 70s which appears more of a 'new' departure. The development of non-prescribing clinic policies and the apparent withdrawal of the medical profession from drug treatment were radical changes. What AIDS has done is to achieve a partial restoration of some of the policy objectives of the pre-1960s situation. Among these objectives was the minimization of harm from drug use, an explicit aim of the 'British System' since the 1920s. The 1926 Rolleston Report enunciated the principle.[27]

When, therefore, every effort possible in the circumstances has been made, and made unsuccessfully, to bring the patient to a condition in which he is independent of the drug, it may . . . become justifiable in certain cases to order regularly the minimum dose which has been found necessary, either in order to avoid serious withdrawal symptoms, or to keep the patient in a condition in which he can lead a useful life.

The mechanisms of policy implementation have changed in the 1980s but the underlying principle remains the same.

Harm-minimization has been defined at two levels – the minimization of harm to the individual drug user, and to society as a whole through prevention of the transmission of the virus. For some commentators, this latter definition appears to be new. Drug policy post-AIDS has been hailed a part of the 'new public health'.[28] But the language of public health in relation to drugs is not new. There is a longstanding tension between preventive and curative approaches, in this as in other areas of health policy. In the nineteenth century, for example, the earlier focus on opium adulteration and child doping and working-class opiate use as part of the public health movement gave place to medical theories of addiction and disease positing individual treatment as the correct option. Nor has 'public health' itself been an unchanging absolute.[29] Its definition and remit has changed in the twentieth century as the nature of state intervention in social issues has itself shifted. The 'new public health' of the 1970s and 80s has much in common with social hygienist views of public health in the early 1900s. Drug policy, both pre- and post-AIDS, with its emphasis on health education, on the role of the voluntary sector, on the drug user as a 'normal' individual responsible for his or her own actions and health, has epitomized key elements of the redefinition. Drugs and public health had been intermittent bed fellows before AIDS – and from a longer-term perspective as well. But despite the intermittent use of the language of public health in relation to drugs and to alcohol, in actual practice drug treatment has remained outside the public health system. Whether AIDS will change that remains to be seen.

One of the key periods of the inter-relationship with public health was in the 1960s, at another time of policy flux. It is instructive to compare the two 'emergency' periods. One commentator has, for example, drawn attention to the parallels between the Advisory Council's part 1 report on AIDS and Drug Misuse and the Brain Committee's report on drug addiction in 1965. Like the ACMD, Brain also justified change in drug policy on public health grounds. Addiction was a 'socially infectious condition', a disease which 'if allowed to spread unchecked, will become a menace to the community'. And the remedies suggested by Brain – including notification and compulsory treatment – were classic public health responses. The balance required in drug policy in the 1980s between minimizing the harm from drug use but not thereby promoting it is paralleled by Brain's attempt to graft the public health objective of preventing infection on to a system geared to individual treatment.[30] Drug doctors had to prescribe opiates to undercut the black market, but not so much that the market was supplied. These are not the only parallels between the 1960s and the 1980s – one can point to an initially enhanced role for research and the social sciences in the 60s and in the 80s; or to the strengthening of the British/American connection in research and policy comparison which has also marked both decades; or even to the revived demands for compulsory treatment as Britain has again moved towards a public health rather than a penal response.

Finally, what has happened to the power relationships within policy post-AIDS? At first sight, AIDS has brought a sea-change. Drugs – common to other areas of health policy, such as alcohol or mental health – have passed from a specialist to a community care model. Needle exchange and the enhanced role of the voluntary agencies offer a non-medical model of service provision. But one enduring theme in drug policy has been that of the relationship between doctors and the state. And, despite the apparent 'demedicalization' of drug policy in the 1980s, in particular post-AIDS, policy making itself appears to have changed little in that respect. After, as before AIDS, it has been exemplified, for example, the influence of doctor civil servants as important in policy making, a theme going back to Dr E. W. Adams, a Ministry of Health civil servant and secretary of the Rolleston Committee in 1924–6, and before him to Dr Norman Kerr, President of the Society for the Study of Inebriety and staunch promoter of the Inebriates Acts from the 1880s. Earlier patterns of medical and other professional involvements have seen a revival through AIDS. In Scotland, the role of the pharmacist in providing free needles has been important, paralleling the profession's nineteenth-century role in dispensing opiates and providing medical care to poor clients.[31] The general practitioner is seen by the ACMD AIDS reports as again having a key role to play, as before the 1960s.

It should perhaps be remembered, too, that Britain, both pre- and post-AIDS, remains part of a national and international system of control which treats drug use as a criminal rather than a health matter. At the international level, such controls have intensified. And domestically attempts to bring the health and criminal justice systems closer together because of the threat of AIDS in prison, as through pre-trial diversion to medical treatment, carry with them the ultimate sanction of compulsory treatment. AIDS may have helped to 'normalize' drug policy at one level. At another, it has served to bind the health and penal aspects of drug control more inextricably than before.

What can we then conclude about the relationship between AIDS, drugs, and history? First that the 'lesson of history' is only invited by policy makers at a time of policy tension and flux, when ways forward are uncertain and the arena seems an open one. In such circumstances, the historian can have a very direct policy input but only at the expense of abandoning the complexities of historical interpretation for a more polemical stance. There was no such role for history in relation to drugs and AIDS in the 1980s, primarily because overall policy objectives were already clear and it suited no policy interest to call on the historical record. The achievement of established policy objectives was better achieved in these circumstances by an emphasis on the newness of developments, as a response to potentially epidemic and unusual circumstances. Stressing previous policy traditions would not have achieved much. But there is, as this essay has argued, a role for history apart from the policy activist one. The more reflective post-crisis period which AIDS policy making has now entered has engendered different thoughts about the role of history. The theme of continuity rather than change in policy has come to the fore – of AIDS itself, and AIDS policy making not as a discontinuity with the past, but as in many respects all of a piece with preceding developments. It is contemporary and near-contemporary developments to which we should turn in order to set the impact of AIDS in proper perspective. Whether the function is that of slow journalism or policy analysis, drug policy in the 1980s and the impact of AIDS must form part of its contemporary history.

ACKNOWLEDGEMENTS

I am grateful to Professor Daniel Fox for comments on an earlier draft of this paper. My thanks are due to the Nuffield Provincial Hospitals Trust for financial support and to Ingrid James for secretarial assistance.

NOTES

This paper originally appeared in a special AIDS issue of the *British Journal of Addiction* and I am grateful to the Editor, Prof. Griffith Edwards, for permission to republish it here.

1 T. McKeown and R. G. Record, 'Reasons for the Decline in Mortality in England and Wales during the Nineteenth Century', in M. W. Flinn and T. C. Smout, eds., *Essays in Social History* (Oxford, 1974).

2 'AIDS: The Public Context of an Epidemic', *Millbank Quarterly*, 64 (1986), Supplement 1; F. Mort, *Dangerous Sexualities: Medico-Moral Politics in England since 1830* (London, 1987); R. Porter, 'Plague and Panic', *New Society*, 12 December 1986, pp. 11–13.

3 A. M. Brandt, *No Magic Bullet. A Social History of Venereal Disease in the United States since 1880 with a New Chapter on AIDS* (New York and Oxford, 1987).

4 J. Austoker, 'AIDS and Homosexuality in Britain: A [*sic*] Historical Perspective', in M. W. Adler, ed., *Diseases in the Homosexual Male* (London, 1988).

5 R. Porter and D. Porter, 'AIDS: Law, Liberty and Public Health', in P. Byrne, ed., *Health, Rights and Resources: Kings College Studies, 1987–8* (London, 1988).

6 R. Porter, 'History says No to the Policeman's Response to AIDS', *British Medical Journal*, 293 (1986), pp. 1589–90.

7 Dorothy Porter, Personal Communication.

8 Social Services Committee, *Third Report from the Social Services Committee. Problems Associated with AIDS*, Vol. 1. Reports and Minutes of Evidence. Memorandum from British Medical Association (London, 1986–7), p. 72.

9 Chief Medical Officer, *On the State of the Public Health. The Annual Report of the Chief Medical Officer of the DHSS for the Year 1986* (London, 1987).

10 For discussion of historians' closer involvement in a policy advisory role, see V. Berridge and P. Strong, 'AIDS, and the Relevance of History', *Social History of Medicine*, 4(1) (1991), pp. 129–38.

11 V. Berridge and P. Strong, 'AIDS Policies in the UK: A Preliminary Analysis', in E. Fee and D. M. Fox, eds., *AIDS: The Making of a Chronic Disease* (Berkeley, 1992).

12 E. Fee and D. M. Fox, 'The Contemporary Historiography of AIDS', *Journal of Social History*, 23(2) (1989), pp. 303–14.

13 For examples of the range of current work and some discussion of developments in historical input, see E. Fee and D. M. Fox, *AIDS: The Burdens of History* (Berkeley, 1988); and E. Fee and D. M. Fox, eds., *AIDS: The Making of a Chronic Disease* (Berkeley, 1992). For discussion of current historical issues around AIDS, see V. Berridge, 'AIDS and the Historian: Conference Report', *Social History of Medicine*, 2(3) (1989).

14 D. M. Fox, P. Day, and R. Klein, 'The Power of Professionalism: AIDS in Britain, Sweden and the United States', *Daedalus* special issue *Living with Aids*, 118(2) (1989).

15 D. P. Adams, 'Wartime Bureaucracy and Penicillin Allocation: The Committee on Chemotherapeutic and Other Agents 1942–44', *Journal of the History of Medicine and Allied Sciences*, 44 (1989), pp. 196–217; W. Muraskin, 'The Silent Epidemic: The Social, Ethical and Medical Problems Surrounding the Fight against Hepatitis B', *Journal of Social History*, 22(2) (1988), pp. 277–98.

16 V. Berridge, 'Drugs and Social Policy: The Establishment of Drug Control in Britain, 1900–1930', *British Journal of Addiction*, 29 (1984), pp. 210–17.

17 T. Duster, *The Legislation of Morality* (New York, 1970); E. Schur, *Narcotic Addiction in Britain and America: The Impact of Public Policy* (London, 1963).

18 D. Musto, *The American Disease: Origins of Narcotic Control* (New Haven and London, 1973).

19 D. T. Courtwright, *Dark Paradise: Opiate Addiction in America before 1940* (Cambridge, Mass., 1982).

20 V. Berridge, 'Historical Issues', in S. MacGregor, ed., *Drugs and British Society* (London, 1989); G. Edwards, 'The British Approach to the Treatment of Heroin Addiction', *Lancet*, 1 (1969), p. 768.

21 D. Downes, *Contrasts in Tolerance: Postwar Penal Policy in the Netherlands and England and Wales* (Oxford, 1988).

22 J. Marks, 'Prescribing Opiates: Who benefits?', *Druglink*, 2(6) (1987), p. 17, repeats the traditional view of the 1920s.

23 Fox, Day, and Klein, 'The Power of Professionalism'.

24 G. Stimson, 'AIDS and HIV: The Challenge for British Drug Services', *British Journal of Addiction*, 85 (1990), pp. 329–39.

25 V. Berridge, 'AIDS and British Drug Policy: History Repeats Itself', in D. Whynes and P. Bean, eds., *Policing and Prescribing: The British System of Drug Control* (London, 1991); G. Stimson, L. Alldritt, K. Dolan, M. Donoghoe, and R. Lart, *Injecting Equipment Exchange Schemes – Final Report* (London, 1988).

26 Advisory Council on the Misuse of Drugs, *Prevention* (London, 1984).

27 Rolleston Report, *Report of the Departmental Committee on Morphine and Heroin Addiction* (London, 1926).

28 G. Stimson and R. Lart, 'HIV, Drugs and Public Health in England: New Words, Old Tunes', *International Journal of Addictions*, 26(12) (1991), pp. 1263–77.

29 J. Lewis, *What Price Community Medicine? The Philosophy, Practice and Politics of Public Health since 1919* (London, 1986).

30 'HIV top priority', says official report, *Druglink*, 3(3) (1988), p. 6.

31 V. Berridge and G. Edwards, *Opium and the People. Opiate Use in Nineteenth Century England* (London, 1987).

ELEVEN

ANOMALIES AND MYSTERIES IN THE 'WAR ON DRUGS'

ANN DALLY

THE non-medical use of drugs today is an example of how society, supported by the medical profession, constructs 'problems' and invents 'diseases' for which they then find 'treatments'. Some pharmacological substances, for example alcohol and tobacco, are major causes of death, yet are permitted to be sold and even advertised, and are a major source of government revenue. Others are regarded as 'ethical', and require a doctor's prescription. Some of the less harmful drugs, for example cannabis and heroin,[1] are made dangerous by myth, politics, illegality, and other social factors. Governments and doctors capitalize on collective fantasies. They publicize the drugs in a way to induce horror and fear. This policy costs governments and nations dearly, but it provides other political benefits, including to the medical profession. The dangers of these substances are both created and emphasized with zeal rather than evidence. Such evidence as exists is liable to be concocted and financed in order to exaggerate their dangers.

Illegal drugs are the subject of a 'phoney war', waged by governments for their own purposes that certainly have nothing to do with the 'dangers' of these substances. Governments who capitalize on public shock-horror have a splendid means of diverting public attention and anger from *real* issues and for interfering in the affairs of other nations, even to the extent of sending spies and troops. This situation is a major cause of crime all over the world and the criminal drug industry is second only to the arms trade in wealth, power, and influence. Whole economies now depend upon the production and sale of illegal drugs and the people who would least like to see the trade decriminalized or legalized are the criminal traders themselves. In no other way could they have so much power or make so much money. This raises a question. How far are governments who purport to make 'war on drugs' actually encouraging, profiting from, and involved in the illegal trade? The same question can be asked of the doctors who support those government policies.

There is little or no evidence that these drugs are in themselves seriously harmful until a political situation leads to the creation of genuinely harmful forms – crack, ecstasy – but there is ample evidence that the harm they do is actually done by the policies constructed round them. Yet few politicians, and only one British politician, have yet admitted this in public. The medical profession accepts and supports government policies and goes along with the idea that drugs, rather than fantasies and policies about drugs, are harming society and must be 'fought'.

For individuals whose fears and fantasies have been stimulated by governments and doctors, the so-called 'drugs crisis' and the 'War on Drugs' is largely a product of what Freud called primary process thinking, i.e. the thinking of fantasy and dreams, unfettered by fact (at least, by fact in context), unimpeded by logic, highly symbolic, and dominated by anomalies and mysteries. My own part in the history of the drugs problem has been largely as a participant and I got into deep trouble as a result, being prosecuted three times by the General Medical Council. This experience has not produced any evidence against my views but it has shown how entrenched are current beliefs about the drugs war and how deeply involved is the medical profession in supporting those beliefs.

The 'War on Drugs' in its many manifestations is being *acted* by doctors, politicians, and public servants who have their own motives, and often behave in ways that are specious, scary, or bizarre. There are few things in the world that damage the quality of life more than present drug policies. These have become so destructive that I suspect that, in the foreseeable future, only historians could sort it out. The present situation depends on people *not* understanding the situation and on maintaining their misbeliefs and prejudices. Much energy and public money is spent on ensuring that this ignorance and misunderstanding continues, along with the shock-horror fantasies that provide essential support for western drug policies.

An historian who starts with a reasonably open mind and a moderate acceptance of the conventional wisdom in the subject is likely to assume that heroin is dangerous, that addiction means inevitable deterioration, that doctors are as honourable towards drug addicts as they are towards other patients, and that America or Britain, or any other country, is reducing or containing the problem rather than *causing* it. Such an historian who looks at the evidence is in for a shock, but it will be a constructive shock.

My interest in drugs was initially clinical, as a practising doctor. I stumbled by chance on something that took me into deep waters.

I began to explore further and came across a situation that certain powerful people did not wish to be explored. They wanted me out of the field, and in the end they got what they wanted, though not, I think, in the way they had intended.

The 'something' on which I stumbled was the discovery that our present situation regarding illegal drugs, including its medical 'treatment', is political and without scientific foundation. Even after thirty years as a practising doctor, I was so shocked by what I found that it destroyed in me last remnants of the youthful idealism that took me into medicine in the first place, when the National Health Service was about to begin and seemed to be a dream come true.

I realized that in scarcely any field is so-called 'truth about drugs' backed by valid evidence. The cooperation of doctors is vital to the politicians and vice versa. In the medical field the evidence for what is done and imposed on others is so feeble as to be virtually non-existent. But important factors are at stake, including the political careers of important people, ambitious doctors, high up civil servants, powerful moralists, and those exploiting less powerful moralists, and, of course, the whole of the world's illegal drugs industry. It is a conspiracy only in the sense that many people and institutions have become involved and now share the need to avoid the truth. It is a dangerous field for an unsuspecting doctor who is simply trying to help patients.

In this situation addicts, whether or not they are also patients, are mostly unable to help themselves. Their self-esteem is low, which is not surprising if one considers how society and the medical profession treat them. It means that they are unable to form a pressure group, even for simply providing information. They still feel they have to play the part of the degraded, dying creatures that society wants them to be. One might say, they are *invented* like that. It is a sad background to the 'War on Drugs' which must be one of the most phoney (or *invented*) wars ever devised or fought. Like many wars, it is based on false information and misinformation, and is basically not really concerned with drugs or drug users.

The first anomaly I am going to mention was actually invented by an historian, Virginia Berridge. With Professor Edwards she wrote a splendid book on opium use in the nineteenth century,[2] published in 1981, when the present so-called 'drugs crisis' was causing concern. There was a visible problem in London and other big cities at the time, due to a sudden change of policy on the part of certain powerful doctors. As a result, addicts, unable to find any help from doctors or anyone else, were congregating in Piccadilly and roaming the streets. Any doctor who was remotely sympathetic was inundated with

potential addict patients begging for help, and was under threat from
the medical establishment. The media were full of shock-horror stories
about drugs. There was a strong need for sensible historical background
information. Yet, in the very first sentence of Berridge and Edwards'
Introduction, we read: 'The most acute anxieties of the 1960s "drug
epidemic" have quietened. Drug stories appear less often, and more
prosaically, in the newspapers.' That statement seems to be a provoca-
tive denial of reality. The rest of the book, about the nineteenth
century, seems to be a model of learning and good sense.

Some of the anomalies in the field of illegal drugs are frankly absurd.
A few months ago I was invited to talk at a provincial medical school
and teaching hospital. I chose the title *Untruths about Heroin are Damaging Civilization*. Notices of the meeting were posted all over the hospital
and university. Mysteriously these spelled the title of my talk as one
word, and they spelled it wrong. It stated that I would talk on

UntruthsaboutHeroinareDamagingCivilization [*sic*]

This word has forty-two letters. Perhaps only the subject of illegal drugs
could produce so absurd a word. No one offered any explanation or
even mentioned it. In matters of drugs, if it is mysterious and incomprehensible, anything goes!

That was not the end of it. I had been particularly careful to make
my talk historical and not to advocate any changes except to call for
more honesty and clarity in the definition of terms. I believe that until
we agree what we are talking about and as long as everyone is talking
about different things, it is impossible to have a reasonable discussion
about drug use, drug dependence, and/or the war on drugs. But as soon
as I had finished I saw that many people had heard a different lecture.
Even the chairman, a retired Professor of Psychiatry, said in his
summing up that I had advocated a free market in heroin. I had not,
but he seemed to find the idea of striving for truth and clarity so
threatening that, so far as he was concerned, I already had heroin on
the supermarket shelves. One person criticized me for, as he put it,
'saying that heroin should be available to expectant mothers'. I had not
mentioned either availability or expectant mothers. Had we been at the
same meeting? I was reassured when several intelligent and relevant
comments and questions made me realize that I was witnessing just
another manifestation of the effect that this extraordinary subject has
on some people.

I told this story while delivering a similar paper at a Wellcome
symposium and again, a member of the audience rose angrily to his feet
and accused me of wishing to put heroin on the supermarket shelves! I

have given versions of that paper on several occasions since. The only time it did *not* elicit a hostile and misheard response was in a small group of sociologists. It seems that the subject of drugs elicits feelings so powerful that some people will always hear falsely. To mishear and distort what is said is the norm in this subject.

The anomalies include the term *narcotic*. The word traditionally refers to drugs named because they aid sleep (though it comes from the Greek *narke*, meaning stiffness or numbness). Yet in illegal drugs, 'narcotics' came to include substances such as amphetamines and cocaine, which are *stimulants*, have the *opposite* effect and actually *prevent* sleep. Even heroin and cannabis are not true narcotics. This has led to confusion. The word 'narcotic' acquired pejorative connotations about substances that were illegal or of which moralists disapproved. It really came to be used to mean 'nasty', 'dangerous', or simply 'illegal'. There are now many different meanings of the word and few attempts to sort them out.

Some drugs, for example opium and its derivatives such as morphine, nepenthe, heroin, were at one time regarded as beneficial to mankind and people kept them and used them rather as they might use aspirin or Valium now. It is interesting that today the image of Valium is beginning to change to something dangerous and sinister. I wonder, will the cycle be repeated?

Somehow the myth arose that so-called 'soft' drugs (whatever those are) are also dangerous. In the term 'soft', most people think of cannabis, which is also illegal but about as harmless as a drug can be – for none are *totally* harmless. It was put about not only that cannabis is dangerous (and all kinds of phoney research was done to 'prove' it) but that it leads to 'hard' drugs such as heroin and cocaine. This must be one of the most politically astute myths of all because it leads to fear, mostly in parents who know nothing about the subject. Yet the connection between 'hard' and 'soft' drugs is that they are both *illegal* and the Dutch have now demonstrated this by separating them in law and showing that the connection no longer exists. I personally asked several hundred heroin addicts what was the connection between cannabis and heroin and their only answer was that if the police seize the available cannabis, dealers offer heroin instead. That was how some of them had become addicted.

Other anomalies: a common Victorian habit, taking a so-called 'narcotic' – opium or cocaine – to relax, which in many could be compared to a couple of pints of beer or a gin and tonic, came to be regarded as a sin and a crime. Addicts, formerly objects of mild disapproval, rather like drunks or smokers today, were gradually turned into criminals and outcasts. This was demonstrated recently in a clever cartoon. The addict Samuel Taylor Coleridge is sitting at his desk writing poetry and smoking opium. Enter the man from Porlock, bowler-hatted, flashing a card. He announces, 'Porlock Drug Squad! You're nicked, Coleridge!'

The virtually universal and fairly harmless custom of taking opium for pain, also came to be regarded as a sin and a crime. Heroin is banned altogether in the US and I have come across some tragic cases in Britain in recent years where people who are dying or have had serious accidents are denied the incomparable benefit of heroin or morphine on the grounds that they might become addicted.

The Harrison Narcotic Act of 1914 in the United States set the scene for the prohibition that has been America's policy ever since. It both reflected and created a climate in which the addict could be reclassified as criminal and morally evil. Britain, or rather British doctors, stood out against American and Home Office efforts to extend the process to Britain. The Rolleston Committee, which reported in 1926, created a liberal, medical, attitude towards drug addiction in what was then a small and largely middle-class problem. This lasted for nearly forty years and enabled many respectable addicts to live normal lives, as they had always been able to do. Some, such as the writer Enid Bagnold, were able to lead prosperous and creative lives while on opiate drugs for as long as sixty years. This gave the lie to the idea that addiction inevitably leads to deterioration, but the evidence, as with other evidence, was ignored or kept secret.

Then, in the 1960s, the system was challenged by an increase in addiction and its extension to that dangerous body, the *working class*. Newspapers began the shock-horror tactics that we know so well. The medical profession changed its attitude and joined the word-abusers and concept-manipulators, even to the extent of allowing, and initiating, shock horror. How did this happen? That is an interesting question and is, I think, important in the history of the medical profession in the twentieth century, though there is no time to explore it here.

In recent years illegal drug use has been given such morally condemnatory labels as 'drug abuse' and 'drug misuse'. These are now regarded as medical *diagnoses*. They appear in official documents and in the names of official bodies – the Advisory Council on the *Misuse* of Drugs is powerful in forming government policy – and incidentally drugs are one of the few subjects about which the two main parties are in complete agreement. There is another government-funded body, the Standing Conference on Drug *Abuse*. Ironically and typically, a new government document emphasizes the importance of not being moralistic about 'drug abuse'![3]

This is the only example I can think of where a *moral judgement* is used as a medical diagnosis. How did this come about? Why does no one, or at least no one with influence, protest? Another way of putting it may be to ask, *In whose interest is this situation maintained?*

The idea of 'drug abuse' as a medical diagnosis, and the attitude it reflects, have produced a language of their own. I call it *Drugspeak*. In George Orwell's *1984* the language Newspeak, the origin of all the modern so-called 'speaks', was designed *in order to make it impossible to think in any way other than the party line.* That's how it is with Drugspeak. Corruption of language is probably inevitable where there are strong reasons for suppressing, confusing, or simply avoiding the truth. It seems that the phrase 'drug abuse', used to mean 'illegal drug use', was first used in the United States to express disapproval of the use of cocaine by Southern blacks. As so often happens, the phrase was, and is, used to condemn the user and his group rather than the drug itself.

The World Health Organization has also tended to attack the user rather than the use of drugs. For instance, one committee said that certain drugs

possess a particular attraction for certain psychologically and socially maladjusted persons who have difficulty in conforming to the usual social norms. These include 'arty' people such as struggling writers, painters, and musicians; frustrated non-conformists; and curious, thrill-seeking adolescents and young adults.

You can work out the details of Drugspeak by looking and listening to the use of such words as 'consensus', 'specialty', 'flexibility', and 'maintenance'. They are all used by drugspeakers in special ways that maintain the *status quo*.

Now another anomaly. In June 1983 the *British Medical Journal* published an article on the treatment of drug addiction that must have broken several barriers or records.[4] For instance, there has long been debate about the scientific value of asking patients about treatment they have had. But data in *this* article were based on asking patients about the treatment that *other patients* had had. I do not think that had ever been done before. Moreover the statistics were absurd or non-existent and the conclusions were *non sequitur*. A lively correspondence followed.[5] One distinguished psychiatrist wrote asking how it was that sixteen and a half addicts had done such and such and said that the article was unworthy of the journal.[6] Another wrote that during his experience of the clinic system which had come into being in 1968, the treatment of addicts became not treatment but a competition between doctors to see who could prescribe the least heroin.[7]

It is a mystery to me that this article was published in the *British Medical Journal*. In 1990, when Peter Bartrip's splendid history of the journal[8] was published, I looked through it for clues. Of course the article was not mentioned, nor was the interesting question about what information can usefully be obtained from patients or from patients talking about other patients. On page 321 the then editor describes how, after 1975, there was 'increased rigour in vetting original articles for publication . . . Initially this means good, unprejudiced and quick peer review, followed by discussion by an editorial committee and statistical assessment.' So what happened here?

That is not the end of the story. A few weeks later that article was used by the General Medical Council, or rather by its prosecuting counsel, against me to show that my treatment of heroin addicts had not conformed to the 'consensus' view. My defence counsel protested (rather too politely, I thought). He pointed out some of the absurdities in the article and quoted the subsequent correspondence. I got the impression that this made no difference to the committee, none of whom, I believe, had any experience of treating addicts. Then, in 1986 and 1987, they used the article against me again. It formed an important part of the opening speech for the prosecution. This time my counsel (a different one) did a brilliant hatchet job on the article and revealed it in all its absurdities. I thought that no one would dare to use it again. It was not mentioned by the GMC for the remainder of my case and their prosecuting counsel did not return to it in his closing speech. But I was wrong. Since then that article has been produced by the GMC prosecutors in every case that I know of against doctors who did not toe the party line in the treatment of heroin addicts. And it is interesting and sad that these prosecutors have mostly got away with it. The reason for this is partly what goes on in the medical defence organizations that organize and pay for doctors' defence. They know and have filed away the fact that the *BMJ* article has been discredited, but they do not mention the fact or produce the evidence unless the doctor concerned mentions it himself, which most of them do not and cannot. It is unlikely that, for example, a busy general practitioner in the provinces will find out this kind of thing unless someone points it out to him. I know personally two doctors who were caught out like this. Both were GPs in the NHS far from London and I have reason to believe that they were two exceptionally good doctors. Their offences were the kind that any well-motivated GP could make any day, and one of them had been set up by the police in a really dirty trick. They were naive enough to trust their advisers and not do much homework. One of them was struck off the Register and the other was suspended for three years. I suspect that had they known what they were up against and had fought yet again the battle about the absurdity of that article, the GMC would not have felt able to impose such harsh punishments. But it does show how, where prejudice and vested interests are involved, such battles have to be fought over and over again. I think it also reveals the corruption of entrenched power.

The story I have just told about the *BMJ* article was largely repeated in the history of the famous or infamous *Guidelines for Good Clinical Practice in the Treatment of Drug Abuse* of 1984 which became known as the *'Misguidelines'*. I have not time to describe here the amazing (and in my view also corrupt) way in which they were drawn up.[9] I was a member of the committee and it was a real eye-opener. The *Guidelines* were immediately used (or misused), and have been ever since, against doctors who disagreed with the official policies. The story of that and many other anomalies is in my book *A Doctor's Story*.

In treatment and administration there are so many anomalies and mysteries that I can give only a few examples. A minor one first, but it is indicative. We are told that the government is anxious to get accurate figures about drug users and that this is important in forming policies. Under the Misuse of Drugs Act, doctors are required to notify the Home Office of every patient they see whom they suspect is using illegal drugs, regardless of whether or not they treat him or prescribe for him. Although I worked in the field for many years I saw little or no evidence of any effort made to inform doctors about this. Most doctors do not even know about it and if they notify addicts at all, it is only when they prescribe a drug on Schedule 1 or 2 of the Misuse of Drugs Act, which, for most doctors, is never. Furthermore, while doctors are paid a small sum for notifying *other* notifiable conditions such as measles, tuberculosis, birth or death, they are not paid for notifying drug addiction. Unless they obtain special labels from the Home Office, they even have to pay for the stamp! It does not seem that the government or the Home Office is very keen to get accurate figures. Why not?

There are many anomalies concerning treatment in Britain's drug dependency clinics. There has never been a proper assessment of the success or failure of these clinics, which were set up in the late sixties in response to political demand and public panic. It is known that various things happen, such as that some patients stay off drugs for six months or more after completing a course of treatment and that some patients go round and round in a seemingly endless cycle of the same treatment programme consisting of treatment, then being theoretically 'drug-free' but actually on the black market, then an 'acknowledged' relapse, then back to the waiting list and more black market. Then another treatment programme, more black market, further relapse, and so on. Because the choice of treatment is so limited (it is marginally greater now because of the AIDS situation) the only option for such a patient is to stay on the black market with all its risks or to repeat the treatment as before. There is a case on record who went through the clinic treatment course twenty-seven times and all he was offered was yet another round.[10] As a practising doctor, I find it hard to decide whether we are in the world of Kafka or the world of Alice in Wonderland. Even harder to understand (or not, depending on how you look at it) are those clinics that make claims like '95% success rate'. Success for *what*? At one time I treated a number of patients who had been in such clinics. All of them had left apparently 'drug-free' but in reality were never off drugs for more than a few days and some not even as long as that. As one addict said, 'If they have a 95% success rate, then I know all the failures twenty times over.'

Who are the patients who attend the clinics? I do not think anyone knows. Studies are done on them as though they are typical of drug addicts in general, or even as if they are *the* population of drug addicts. They are not. The Home Office itself has reckoned that it knows at most about only one addict in five, 20%. Of these less than one in three is ever seen at a clinic, say 6% of the total. Of these only a proportion stay on for treatment – half would probably be overstating it. That is 3%. Of those only a small proportion complete the course, some would say less than 1% of those who *attend* – making 0.03% of the total, but even if we are generous and put it at 50%, that's still only 1.5% of all addicts. And most of these relapse within a year or two. So why do they talk in terms of 'success' and what are doctors doing trying to treat them all by the standard, official, routine, or the current 'flexible' regime, with its narrow choice of options?

When I was trying to learn about drug addiction and was puzzling out what on earth was going on, I visited three clinics. In theory all were fully booked with patients. At that time the clinics were crying out for new funds to alleviate the rising tide of addiction and the intolerable burden of patients. In two of these clinics not a single patient turned up. The doctors and other staff waited for a couple of hours, then went home. The third clinic I visited was specially for addicts who were in trouble with the courts. They were being considered for treatment as an alternative to going to prison. They all turned up and were really eager. Each patient was asked whether he was genuine in his desire for treatment or whether he was just trying to avoid going to prison? They all said that it was *nothing* to do with the court case and that they *genuinely* wished for treatment. They were all accepted. Later I heard from a number of patients who had been through the course that drugs circulated freely in the hospital ward and that a patient could get anything he wanted. The staff turned a blind eye and recorded as a 'cure' anyone who was not actually caught with drugs. This satisfied the hospital figures. It satisfied the court. And it satisfied the addicts.

When I was treating drug addicts I always used to write to their former clinics for reports on them as is the custom in clinical medicine. Normally (i.e. with patients who are not 'drug' cases) you get a useful report or summary of the case. But not here. Clinics usually sent many bulky pages of photocopied material from the patient's notes, usually giving an enormous amount of irrelevant information such as recordings of normal blood pressure over many years (incidentally another anomaly is the concentration of many drug dependency 'experts' on normal blood pressure; I have never been able to find out why they do this). But these reports nearly always omitted what I thought was important, for example, the psychiatric assessments of the patient and the doses of drugs prescribed over the years. I do not believe that psychiatric assessments had ever been done in many cases, and the information about their drugs was often withheld, even if I wrote again for it. I came to the conclusion that it was related to the change of prescribing policies in the clinics which occurred in the late 1970s. They suddenly changed from prescribing more or less what the patient asked for as long as he wanted it to prescribing much smaller doses for only a few weeks and then recording the patient as 'drug-free', while at the same time trying to impose the new regime on all doctors. Yet only a few years before they had been prescribing huge doses, up to twenty times more than the doses they were now saying were acceptable.

Another anomaly was that if the clinics sent the information about doses at all, it usually concerned only what was *officially* prescribed. Mention was often made of how the patient had 'reduced' his dose, but hardly ever of the fact that as a result he was now using black market heroin, though you mostly only had to look at his arm to see this. Strangely, the clinic notes kept all sorts of information, like that on blood pressure, which I thought relatively unimportant, yet usually did not record the patient's black market habits, which I thought were very important. They were *all* on the black market so it seemed to me dishonest to record them as being 'drug-free' just because they no longer received *prescribed* drugs.

This sudden change of prescribing policy is another anomaly. Why did it happen? It is often said to be based on a study of prescribing for addicts long term versus short term, published in the Archives of General Psychiatry in 1980, several years *after* the change. That research is often said to show that short-term prescribing and refusing the addict more than a small minimum is better than long-term prescribing and that prescribing injectable drugs to those who are going to use them anyway is counter-productive. I do not want to go into the details of these arguments about doses and injection and so on. In theory they are at the heart of the dispute but I believe that basically they are moral questions which people try to prop up with figures acquired or arranged in ways that suit their beliefs. In fact it is difficult to see the results of that study. It was quite short and if anything the figures seem to indicate the *opposite* of what it was later said to have said. This study is widely used, so widely that now, more than fifteen years after the change, it is still used as the basis for the anti-prescribing argument. So is another study that has an even more chequered history. A research worker studied addicts in their then customary habitat, Piccadilly Circus, and published an article indicating that those who had long-term prescriptions from doctors did better than those without. Then the same author published another article using the same material but coming to the *opposite* conclusion. I was told by someone who knows these things that the first article did not please those in power. Whatever the explanation, it does suggest that figures, like Humpty Dumpty, can mean what you want them to mean, no more, no less.

I spent many hours in libraries puzzling over things like that and I was unable to understand what the so-called 'evidence' indicated. It was a long time before I realized, and actually a high-up Home Office official pointed it out to me, that there simply was not any valid 'evidence' to support the way patients were treated. It was all personal and political. Only then did the whole thing begin to make sense.

Much could be said about the effects of all this and about the world drug situation. The crime. The wrecking of lives. The degeneration and hounding of potentially useful human beings. But I should like briefly to mention one result of western drug policies, *corruption*, because that is perhaps the biggest anomaly of all. Corruption is built into the policies, both the law enforcement policies and the medical policies. When it is uncovered it is often attributed to the drugs, but really it is due to the drug *policies*. It affects everyone in the drugs field, addicts, drug enforcement officers, civil servants, policemen, doctors. I could give you many examples of all these but I shall confine myself to few. In just one American state, Georgia, over a period of five years, thirty-two sheriffs were jailed for drugs offences.[11] What can you expect when, for instance, a police chief is offered half a million dollars to be in church on a particular Sunday morning and another the same sum *not* to be anywhere near the local airfield, where he probably would not be going anyway? The inevitable corruption is not only of those caught by the law but of those who administer the law and those who work under it. I believe it is the *worst* aspect of the 'War on Drugs'.

An example of corruption in Britain (and I could give you many examples) is the number of policemen, especially in London, who have been found guilty during the past few years of drug offences, mostly selling drugs or planting them on people whom they then charge with 'possession with intent to supply', a weasel charge. I have personally come across many cases of police corruption, but none of those led to charges. I believe that this corruption of police has been influential in lowering public regard for the police and it may have contributed to the generally low standards which have led to recent police scandals involving other forms of crime.

The corruption of doctors makes me, as a doctor, particularly sad. When the present drug problems began to surface, in the early 1960s, I believe we could have contained it by encouraging general practitioners to help addicts, perhaps for extra payment, and psychiatrists could have been available to deal with difficult cases. But we did not do that. The government of the day wanted to make a more dramatic show, the public wanted to see more action, and some doctors in what were regarded as rather inferior backwaters (such as the old asylums) wanted more power. So we got expensive clinics that were shut away from the GPs and even from the hospitals where they were placed. Other departments in the hospital were not and are not interested. They do not want to see addicts and do not care what happens to them. The clinics are isolated and the normal system of checks and balances between departments does not operate in them. Other doctors got the idea that *all* drug cases need specialist treatment, though this is no more true in drug addiction than in anything else. Drug addiction was pushed into corners where new so-called 'specialists' carved out careers. GPs ceased to regard it as anything to do with them and developed an antipathy to it. I once did a survey of eighteen GPs in an outer suburb of London to find out whether they would consider treating addicts, which, in theory, they are officially encouraged to do. The official line on this has long been verbally to encourage GPs to look after addicts while at the same time discouraging them by covert threats. Some GPs now even believe, or choose to believe, that they are not *allowed* to treat addicts, which is quite untrue. Anyway, of my eighteen GPs, not one was willing to look after addicts and sixteen were positively hostile to the idea. Some GPs even put up notices saying that they will not treat drug addicts even for conditions unrelated to drugs. Although this is against the terms of their contracts, none has ever been disciplined for refusing to treat a drug addict. It seems that addicts attract a kind of 'licensed nastiness' wherever they go and no one cares about them. A few addicts have complained to the GMC, but they always get the same answer – that the GMC 'has no power' in such matters! Even worse, some GPs refuse to treat the families of drug addicts. I have often had to act as unofficial GP to wives and children, even for tiny babies. It was really upsetting. It is as though people are now programmed to think that everyone with any connection with drug addicts is untouchable and to be rejected. That is a dangerous belief in a doctor.

Yet the former Chief Inspector of Drugs at the Home Office, Bing Spear, who probably knows more about the problem than anyone else in the country, has often been quoted as saying that at the time the panic about drugs began and the law was changed, 'We didn't need clinics. We needed a thousand doctors to take on one addict each.'[12] I have heard him say it many times. Had that happened, I believe that the problem of drugs and treatment by GPs would have developed together and much more healthily. Britain was in a situation from which she might have led the world but she threw away the chance. Now that is all water under the bridge. Fortunately things have begun to improve and a small but increasing number of GPs now do look after the addicts on their lists.

Another anomaly is that it seems that at the time no one except the politicians both medical and general even *wanted* the clinics. Some hospitals had to be bribed, for example, with research money, to create them, and even then some of them took the money and then did not build the clinics.[13] The papers are now being released under the thirty-year rule. I heard that some of them have mysteriously disappeared but I am sure there is plenty of material left there for a perceptive historian.

Then there is the corruption of the law itself, the erosion of human rights, at first applied only in situations of drug 'abuse' or drug trafficking but then extended to wider situations (for example, in the Criminal Justice Acts, and for fraud). It seems to be generally accepted now that a person found guilty of selling drugs is assumed to have obtained all his assets illegally and these can be confiscated by law unless he can prove his innocence. The principle that a person is deemed to be guilty until proved innocent is new in British law, though some might say it already existed in immigration. Since people are taught to hate and despise drug addicts and people do not care much what happens to those they hate and despise, no one protests. If a politician wishes to limit liberty and human rights, it is a good way to do it. I think that needs to be looked into too.

The existence of drugs lowers environmental standards (or 'the quality of life'). In international affairs, particularly American foreign policy, strongly supported by Britain, drugs provide a splendid excuse to interfere in the affairs of foreign countries (Colombia, Central America, Pakistan) or to resist international cooperation (Thatcher's attitude to abolishing European frontier control). Are such power games the nub of the whole extraordinary business? Is the situation an exercise in using people's fears and prejudices in order to increase political power? What other possible explanations are there?

Bias, misinformation, and vested interests are now so entrenched that it is impossible to have open discussions about illegal drugs until those taking part agree on the meaning of the terms. Even then, there is so much prejudice and fear that it is likely to be impossible. Thus discourse about whether or not 'narcotics' should be legalized or 'decriminalized' has little meaning at present.

It is sometimes forgotten that drug addicts are mostly basically normal people, with normal problems and families, jobs, and aspirations. I have collected three albums of photographs of families and children and holidays and hobbies.[14] Each concerns a drug addict or the children of a drug addict. It shows them getting married, playing with their children, boating, birdwatching and so on.

An important prop for maintaining the 'War on Drugs' has been the government campaign against drug use. It began with posters as well as TV. The posters were of the actor who became a 'pin-up' boy because of his effect on teenagers. It continued on TV mostly after midnight when most addicts are in bed like anyone else. Advertisements are trying to sell us something. We know that it is to warn against heroin, to counteract heroin, to urge us not to take it. Yet it is a campaign based on lies and targeting a specific group. A white male, good-looking in the modern style – he became a pin-up. Is the campaign directed at the white, trendy community? If he did not take drugs he could be you or your son. The implication is that if he had not been so foolish as to 'choose' drugs – or if he had not *failed* to 'just say no', he would have been a presentable chap. It is *only* the drugs that prevent him from being 'one of us'.

This reinforces fears and prejudices of the well-defended. The only black in the group of posters I managed to get was the porter pushing the trolley, emphasizing his low status occupation. Seemingly the campaign was trying not to offend the black community by associating drugs with ethnicity and also making a point of not associating it with housing, unemployment, poverty, etc. The whole campaign seemed to aim to induce smugness in a targeted group who would probably never touch drugs. There is a cosy feeling about being told what you 'know' is true.

The campaign also aimed to maintain widespread untruths about heroin. The advertisement assumed that we know that you get 'low' if you take heroin. It compounds this with 'How low can you get?' There is no room for asking 'Do you get low?' or even 'Why do you get low?' It offers no evidence. Of what it actually says, only the constipation is true. The aching limbs go with *withdrawal* from the drug, but if you are going to confuse the effects of heroin with the effects of withdrawal, why mention only this? Much worse are the diarrhoea, anxiety, severe pain, and so on.

The lies mean that the advertisements lose credibility with anyone who knows anything about drugs. The campaign assumes that the 'just say no' approach is easy. Every addict knows it is easy only for people who are not tempted. There is no mention of *nutrition* or the fact that heroin addicts get ill not because they take drugs (unless they take too much, as with alcohol or any other drug) but because they spend all their money on drugs and do not eat properly. There is no mention of *poisons* – the dangers of shooting into your veins the impurities with which black market drugs are cut: brick dust, Vim, flour, and so on. These and not the drug itself are what damages. Every addict knows this so obviously the campaign is not directed at them. Those who have any contact with drug users know it too. These include the young people likely to be recruited to drugs, just the people, you would think, that the government want to influence. But by telling them lies, the authorities lose any credibility they might have had. The only people likely to be impressed are those who know nothing about drugs and are unlikely to come into contact with them. It is their prejudices that this campaign aims to reinforce. They are probably the majority (or thought to be the majority) and they have many votes. Presumably these are the audience that is being targeted.

It seems to me that the classification made in the government anti-drug campaign is between drug takers who are white, foolish, and simply fail to say 'no' and non-drug users who are white and have had the sense to 'just say no'. It is a way of targeting a group who already believe what you are saying, to make them feel more secure and perhaps smug, and to give the appearance that you are tackling a serious problem.

One of the difficulties in the history of medicine is to see modern situations and constructions in as detached and critical a way as we see past situations. The present situation in drugs, if you bother to examine the evidence, is a wonderful opportunity to do just that.

NOTES

1 H. Dale Beckett, 'Heroin: The Gentle Drug', *New Society*, 26 July 1979.
2 Virginia Berridge and G. Edwards, *Opium and the People. Opiate Use in Nineteenth Century England* (London, 1981).
3 Reported in *Independent* newspaper, 17 December 1991.
4 T. Bewley and A. H. Ghodse, 'Unacceptable Face of Private Practice: Prescription of Controlled Drugs to Addicts', *British Medical Journal*, 286 (1983), pp. 1876–7.
5 R. Hartnoll and R. Lewis, Letter, *British Medical Journal*, 287 (1983), p. 500.
6 Peter Dally, Letter, *British Medical Journal*, 287 (1983), p. 500.
7 James H. Willis, Letter, *British Medical Journal*, 287 (1983), p. 500.
8 Peter Bartrip, *Mirror of Medicine: A History of the BMJ* (Oxford, 1990).
9 Ann Dally, *A Doctor's Story* (London, 1990), chapter 9.
10 Information given by H. B. Spear when he was Chief Inspector of Drugs to the Home Office, c. 1986.
11 Prof. J. Killorin, Personal Communication based on local statistics.
12 H. B. Spear, formerly Chief Inspector of Drugs, Home Office, Personal Communication.
13 A. Baker, former Senior Medical Officer, Ministry of Health, Personal Communication.
14 Now lodged in the Contemporary Medical Archive Collection at the Wellcome Institute for the History of Medicine, London.

GLOSSARY

AIDS: acquired immuno deficiency syndrome due to infection by the
    human immuno deficiency virus (HIV)
AZT: abbreviation for 3'-azido-2', 3'-dideoxythymidine, a drug used in
    the treatment of AIDS
laudanum: a preparation containing opium
liniment: a liquid preparation, applied externally to the skin
mithridatium: a substance believed to be a remedy against any poison
paregoric: a remedy containing camphorated opium
spirit of hartshorn: ammonia
theriac: antidote to the bite of venomous animals

INDEX

'Abbas I, shah of Iran, 35
'absorption theory' (of action of opium),
    58–9, 60, 70
acacia, 9, 16–17
Acheson, Sir Donald, 189
Adams, Dr E. W., 195
Adams, Samuel Hopkins, 117–18, 119
addiction, 2, 18, 119, 200; as criminal
    matter, 191–2, 196, 203–4; as disease,
    121, 191, 194, 204; iatrogenic, 114, 117,
    121, 122–3, 126–7, 129 n. 12; treatment,
    121, 122, 123, 191, 195, 196, 205–9,
    211–12; see also addicts; clinics; opium
addicts: attitudes of doctors towards, 201–2,
    211–12; perceptions of, 121, 123–4,
    126–7, 160, 194, 203–4, 212–13;
    self-image, 121, 201
advertisements, 119, 120, 164, 213–14
Advisory Council on the Misuse of Drugs
    (ACMD), 194, 195, 196, 204
Africa, 26, 157, 180, 188
AIDS, historical consciousness surrounding,
    187–96
Alaska natives, 133
alchemy, 28, 29, 31
alcohol, 28, 35, 199; see also alcoholism;
    beer; distilled liquor; Navajo Indians;
    women
alcoholism, 31, 157; treatment, 147, 152
Alexis I, tsar of Russia, 34
alkaloids, 170, 176; isolation of, 62, 116,
    169; see also opium
Allen, William, 169
Allen & Hanburys, 169, 171, 172–3, 176,
    177, 179, 183
Almeida, J., 28
almond-oil, 13, 14
Alpini, Prosper, 27
Alston, Charles, 55–6, 57, 63, 64
'alum curds', 14
Amazonian Indians, use of cacao, 26

America, tobacco cultivation, 33; see also
    United States
American Bar Association, 191
American Druggist and Pharmaceutical Record,
    163, 164
American Medical Association (AMA),
    114, 115, 118–19, 120, 122–3, 124, 191;
    Council on Pharmacy and Chemistry,
    115–16, 119, 120, 121
American Pharmaceutical Association,
    165
American United Drug Company, 177
amphetamines, 203
Amsterdam, 27, 40, 42, 44
anaesthetics, 178, 180
analgesic, see opium
Anatolia, coffeehouses in, 40
Andreas (d. 217 BC), discussion of opium, 5,
    6
Andromachus the Elder, 17
Andromachus the Younger, 17
animal experimentation, 53–60, 62, 63–4;
    ethical aspects, 68–9, 70; transferability of
    findings to humans, 65
Anna of Austria, queen of France, 42
antibiotics, 181
Antifebrine, 98
Antipyrine, 99, 103, 108 n. 13, 171
Apache Indians, 136, 137, 147; San Carlos
    and Whiteriver, 137
aphrodisiacs, 29, 30, 31, 35
apothecaries, 30, 31, 32; English, 77, 79; see
    also chemists; pharmacists
Arab medicine, 31
Armenian merchants, 27
Arsenic Act (1851), 94, 95
arsenical compounds, 115, 175–6, 178
arsenobenzol-billon, 175
Asclepiades, 6, 19 n. 20
Asia, 26, 35, 42
aspirin, 171, 175

217